A
Sacred Covenant

The Spiritual Ministry
of Nursing

A
Sacred Covenant

The Spiritual Ministry
of Nursing

Mary Elizabeth O'Brien, SFCC,
PHD, MTS, RN, FAAN

The Catholic University of America
School of Nursing
Washington, DC

JONES AND BARTLETT PUBLISHERS
Sudbury, Massachusetts
BOSTON   TORONTO   LONDON   SINGAPORE

World Headquarters

Jones and Bartlett Publishers
40 Tall Pine Drive
Sudbury, MA 01776
978-443-5000
info@jbpub.com
www.jbpub.com

Jones and Bartlett Publishers
Canada
6339 Ormindale Way
Mississauga, Ontario L5V 1J2
CANADA

Jones and Bartlett Publishers
International
Barb House, Barb Mews
London W6 7PA
UK

Jones and Bartlett's books and products are available through most bookstores and online booksellers. To contact Jones and Bartlett Publishers directly, call 800-832-0034, fax 978-443-8000, or visit our website, www.jbpub.com.

Substantial discounts on bulk quantities of Jones and Bartlett's publications are available to corporations, professional associations, and other qualified organizations. For details and specific discount information, contact the special sales department at Jones and Bartlett via the above contact information or send an email to specialsales@jbpub.com.

The authors, editor, and publisher have made every effort to provide accurate information. However, they are not responsible for errors, omissions, or for any outcomes related to the use of the contents of this book and take no responsibility for the use of the products and procedures described. Treatments and side effects described in this book may not be applicable to all people; likewise, some people may require a dose or experience a side effect that is not described herein. Drugs and medical devices are discussed that may have limited availability controlled by the Food and Drug Administration (FDA) for use only in a research study or clinical trial. Research, clinical practice, and government regulations often change the accepted standard in this field. When consideration is being given to use of any drug in the clinical setting, the health care provider or reader is responsible for determining FDA status of the drug, reading the package insert, and reviewing prescribing information for the most up-to-date recommendations on dose, precautions, and contraindications, and determining the appropriate usage for the product. This is especially important in the case of drugs that are new or seldom used.

Library of Congress Cataloging-in-Publication Data
O'Brien, Mary Elizabeth.
 A sacred covenant : the spiritual ministry of nursing / Mary Elizabeth O'Brien.
   p. ; cm.
 Includes bibliographical references and index.
 ISBN 978-0-7637-5571-3 (alk. paper)
 1. Nursing—Religious aspects—Christianity. 2. Nursing ethics. 3. Nurse and patient. 4. Spirituality. I. Title.
 [DNLM: 1. Nurse-Patient Relations. 2. Spirituality. 3. Christianity. 4. Nursing Care. WY 87 O13sa 2008]
 RT85.2.O3694 2008
 261.8'32173--dc22
                              2007045874
6048

Production Credits
Executive Editor: Kevin Sullivan
Aquisitions Editor: Emily Ekle
Associate Editor: Amy Sibley
Editorial Assistant: Patricia Donnelly
Production Director: Amy Rose
Associate Production Editor: Amanda Clerkin
Associate Marketing Manager: Rebecca Wasley
Manufacturing and Inventory Control Supervisor: Amy Bacus
Composition: Shawn Girsberger
Cover Design: Kristin E. Ohlin
Cover Image Credit: © Dawn Hudson/ShutterStock, Inc.
Interior Icon Credit: © Cyrill Kourachov/ShutterStock, Inc.
Printing and Binding: Malloy, Inc
Cover Printing: Malloy, Inc.

Printed in the United States of America
11 10 09 08 07   10 9 8 7 6 5 4 3 2 1

Dedication

For all nurses who lovingly embrace a sacred covenant of caring in their ministry to the ill and the infirm.

Author's Note

The scripture quotations contained herein are from the *New Revised Standard Version Bible: Catholic Edition,* copyright © 1993 and 1989 by the Division of Christian Education of the National Council of Churches of Christ in the U.S.A. Used by permission. All rights reserved.

Contents

Introduction

Ever since being introduced to the spiritual and theological understanding of "covenant" during participation in an Old Testament course, I have wanted to explore the concept in relation to the spirituality of nursing. My personal clinical nursing and nursing research experiences had hinted that unique and deeply spiritual bonds are formed during nurse–patient interactions. Thus I wanted to further explore these relationships as experienced by other practicing nurses.

During the past few years I have collected a multiplicity of caregiving anecdotes from nurses ministering in a variety of settings; these have well validated the "sacredness" of the covenantal bonding between nurses and their patients. Some dimensions of the sacred nursing covenant discussed in this book include: being called with a "holy calling," "ministers of a new covenant," a "tradition of service," "entering sacred spaces," "committed to caring," "blessed vulnerability," "empowered by faith," and the "mysticism of everyday nursing."

Concepts discussed in *A Sacred Covenant* are grounded in biblical passages taken from both Old and New Testament scripture. Each chapter begins with a scripturally oriented nursing meditation and ends with a biblically themed nurse's prayer; these may be used either individually or in groups.

Chapter 1 explores the spiritual ministry of nursing as a sacred covenant focusing on the nurse's being called by name, service to others, and the nurse as "God's flute." In Chapter 2 the spirituality of caregiving is explored in terms of nursing ministry, including such concepts as entering "deep water," bringing "good news" to patients, and caring for the sick as described in *Matthew* 25:36–40. Chapter 3 examines the spiritual history of nursing reflected in the "tradition of service" and "varieties of gifts" possessed by nurses; love, strength, and commitment are nursing virtues highlighted. In Chapter 4 the gift of nursing compassion is discussed in relation to such concepts as healing, holy ground, and gentleness, and Chapter 5 describes a nurse's compassion in examining commitment to caring as supported by God's steadfast love. Chapter 6 explores the nurse's vulnerability, and Chapter 7, the nurse's faith. Finally, Chapter 8 explores the "hidden ministry of nursing" within the framework of the "mysticism of everyday nursing."

In each chapter anecdotes shared by practicing nurses are used to illustrate the spiritual themes as lived practically within the mysticism of everyday nursing. Pseudonyms are used, for both patients and nurses, wherever naming is warranted.

I wish to express special thanks to Kevin Sullivan, Amy Sibley, Amanda Clerkin, and Kristin Ohlin, of Jones and Bartlett Publishers, for carefully and enthusiastically taking on the task of shepherding the manuscript to publication.

Ultimately, I am deeply grateful to God for the blessing of being His "flute" in the sharing of powerful and poignant stories that reflect the sacred covenant of nursing. I give thanks to the Father who provides the strength and courage to write, to His Divine Son whose passionate commitment to caring inspires my work, and to the Holy Spirit without whose inspiration these pages would never come to light.

1 ☽ A Sacred Covenant: The Spiritual Ministry of Nursing

I will establish my covenant with you.

Genesis 6:18

THE SACRED COVENANT OF CARING

Gentle God,
  Who blessed the world with
    A holy covenant of love,
  You have called Your nurses
    To a sacred covenant of caring:

A sacred covenant of compassionately
  serving ill brothers and sisters;

A sacred covenant of tenderly comforting
  anxious brothers and sisters;

A sacred covenant of kindly encouraging
  elder brothers and sisters;

A sacred covenant of gently nurturing
  younger brothers and sisters;

A sacred covenant of caringly protecting
  mentally challenged brothers and sisters;

A sacred covenant of solicitously guarding
  homeless brothers and sisters;

and,

A sacred covenant of lovingly supporting
dying brothers and sisters.

Bless, Dear Lord, this sacred covenant of
caring, to which You have
called Your nurses.

Help us to be worthy!

I recently began one of my classes on "Spirituality in Nursing" with a meditation on the beautiful prayer of the great Saint Teresa of Avila, "Christ Has No Body Now But Yours." In the prayer Saint Teresa reminds us that because our Lord no longer walks the earth in human form, it is we, His followers, who must carry out His ministry of healing.

What a magnificent teaching this is for nurses! How blessed we are in our vocation of caring to realize that we can be used by Jesus as messengers of His love. It is our eyes that the Lord can use to look with compassion on the world. It is our feet that He can use to carry His healing grace to the ill and the infirm. It is our hands that He can use to touch with His tenderness those who are suffering and in pain. The choice and the commitment, made by nurses, to be used by Jesus as His ministers to the sick may be envisioned as a "sacred covenant," as a lived experience of the spiritual ministry of nursing.

At the beginning of time God gave us an incredible gift in promising to establish a covenant with His people. We all love to receive promises, especially when it comes to personal relationships, associations that have become so fragile in contemporary society. In describing His relationship with humankind as a "covenant," the Lord added a strong and unique spiritual dimension to His bond of caring and commitment. God was guaranteeing that His love is real, continuous, and unending.

God's covenantal bonding, as described by spiritual writer Henri Nouwen, provides a sensitive and powerful undergirding for the nurse-patient relationship. Nouwen observed, "In a covenant there is no condition put on faithfulness. It is the unconditional commitment to be of service."[1]

Have we nurses not frequently experienced satisfaction and even joy over patient interactions that may have tested our living out of the concepts of "faithfulness" and "unconditional commitment to be of service"? It is often precisely in patient care situations that stretch our caring and compassion that nurses find the heart of their blessed vocation to serve the ill and the infirm.

When I was first introduced, in an Old Testament course, to the meaning of God's covenant with His people, I began exploring the concept as a model for the nurse's relationship with his or her patients. The term *covenant*, "an important and recurring theme in scripture," describes God's relationship with such Old Testament figures as Noah, Abraham, Moses, and David; the relationship "grows progressively richer in promise until the coming of Christ ushers in the 'new covenant.' "[2] This understanding of the meaning of God's covenant well reflects the spirit of the nurse–patient relationship: "God takes the initiative; this is not agreement between equal parties. God draws up the terms. He makes them known. And He alone guarantees their keeping."[3]

In the relationship between nurse and patient, it is indeed the nurse who must take the initiative; he or she has control in terms of caring behaviors. Although the patient can, of course, ask questions and make requests, it is essentially the nurse who "draws up the terms," who sets the parameters of the relationship. And, it is the nurse who must guarantee the "keeping" of the covenant, for a patient, in the midst of illness and suffering, may need support and guidance in maintaining the therapeutic relationship.

Ultimately, nurses' covenants with their patients, especially those covenants that model the sacredness of God's covenant with His people, are derived from the nurse's calling, from a holy calling.

CALLED WITH A HOLY CALLING

> *Join with me...relying on the power of God, who saved us and called us with a holy calling, not according to our works but according to His own purpose and grace.*
>
> 2 Timothy 1:8–9

How blessed a gift we have, as nurses, to be "called with a holy calling." Nursing is not only a respected profession, it is a beautiful and holy vocation. Caring for the sick is not only a job, it is a ministry, a ministry to the weakest, the neediest, the most fragile of our brothers and sisters in the human family. It is a ministry named by Jesus Himself as one of the primary works of His public life as well as a ministry for those who would follow Him.

Healing of the sick was such an important and holy task for the Lord that He allowed even a person who only touched the hem of His garment to be cured. In the act of caring, of healing, Jesus not only touched those who were suffering but He allowed himself to be touched by them that they might feel the power of His love. And from the Lord's healing came also the ill person's salvation.

Jesuit Jerome Neyrey identifies the above scripture passage, describing a "holy calling" as reflecting the "Pauline model of vocation," commenting, "Paul recalls that his vocation was a gift of God's grace";[4] "this grace," he adds "was already active 'before time began' which is a typical Jewish statement about pre-eminence which stresses how holy or important something is."[5]

From the inception of Christian ministry to those who are ill, as carried out by the earliest followers of Jesus, nursing the sick was considered a holy calling. Nurse historian M. Patricia Donahue points out that because of Jesus' mandate to initiate such ministerial activities as feeding the hungry, giving drink to the thirsty, welcoming strangers, and caring for the ill (as reported in the Gospel of *Matthew* 25:35), "a spiritual meaning became deeply attached to the care of the sick and suffering."[6] "This flowering of Christian idealism," Donahue adds, "was to forever have a deep and significant impact upon the practice of nursing."[7] Ultimately, because of Jesus' own witness in healing the ill and the disabled as well as teaching His disciples to go and do likewise, early Christians saw "caring for the sick (as) an activity especially pleasing to God and (a ministry) through which an individual might inherit 'eternal life.'"[8]

Writing in 1920, pioneer nurse historians Lavinia Dock and Isabel Stewart also described the holiness of the nurse's calling as related directly to the teachings of Jesus: "The disciples' love for their great Teacher took the instant form of service to whomever needed it, especially the sick, neglected and destitute."[9] As Dock and Stewart observed: "Christ's own parables and miracles had dealt much with disease and death, and He told His followers that in ministering to the poor and the sick they were ministering to Him."[10] An important dimension of the new Christian faith was "'not to be ministered unto, but to minister,'" and in later years, "the Golden Rule was often carved on the seats of hospitals."[11]

In 1851, Florence Nightingale admitted that she had, since she was a child, "thought God had called" her to nurse the sick.[12] Miss Nightingale wrote in a note to her first student-nurse probationers, "Our Heavenly Father thanks you for what you do. Lift high the royal banner of nursing. Christ is the author of our profession."[13] It is also reported that when Florence Nightingale was first presented with a suggestion that the nursing profession should be regulated through registration, she replied that nursing "could not be organized like a trade union, nursing was a sacred calling."[14]

Megan, a home care nurse, described the "holiness" of her calling in relating the story of caring for 65-year-old Mr. McMullen, who was homebound as the result of a recurrent glioblastoma. Meg described Mr. McMullen as "unable to walk" and needing help with all activities of daily living; he was also aphasic as a result of his tumor and surgery. Nevertheless, Megan reported that Mr. McMullen's spirituality made it a joy to care for him: "It was such an amazing inspiration to me, to see him remain so positive, and totally full of hope for his future with God." Mr. McMullen's illness progressed, however, and Meg admitted, "I became quite attached to Mr. McMullen and I was not eagerly anticipating our final visit together. He had become like an old friend; he challenged my faith and opened my eyes to a higher level of devotion. When I asked him how he did it, how he managed to keep such a positive spirit when he had deteriorated so much physically ... he looked at me and smiled and told me that it was simple. Love surrounded him, love filled him and remained in him all the time."

Meg added, "Mr. McMullen said that he was totally at peace knowing that God was love, and His love was perfect. I had never considered it in this context before and found myself reflecting for days on the beauty of my interactions with Mr. M., on the holiness of my calling and I thanked God for the gift of my nursing."

Over and over, in the following pages, nurses' reports reflecting the holiness of their calling are repeated. Not all anecdotes describe such inspiring attitudes and behaviors as that of Meg's patient, Mr. McMullen. Nevertheless, myriad records of powerful and profound nurse–patient interactions, elicited through many hours of listening to nurses' stories of caring, demonstrate clearly and unequivocally the blessing and the beauty of the nurse's "holy calling" to care for the sick.

CALLED BY NAME

But now thus says the Lord, he who created you ... Do not fear, for
I have redeemed you; I have called you by name, you are mine.

Isaiah 43:1

Names are very important to us, our own names especially. A name may suggest several things about an individual such as gender, ethnic background (especially surnames), general age category (few older women are named Tiffany or Amber), and possibly even religious affiliation (Sarah and Rebekah, traditionally Jewish women's names, and Mary and Anne, names often given to Roman Catholic girls). Names may also honor an older or deceased family member such as a parent or grandparent. Most of us are proud of our names. They represent who we are and proclaim something about us to those we meet.

Thus when someone significant in our lives, such as a teacher, a minister, or a new friend, "calls us by name" it generally arouses pleasure and a sense of relationship. We like knowing that we are important enough in the eyes of that person that he or she knows our name and can call it when we interact. How much more powerful then is it to realize that the loving God who created us has also "called us by name" and promised that we belong to Him. We are, to God, not simply another member of the large family of humankind that He created. No, each one of His children is so special and unique that we are, in fact, "called by name" to live out our particular vocations as ministers of His love and caring.

An earlier discussion described the overall "holy calling" of nursing, but what does it mean for an individual to be "called by name" to be a nurse? Perhaps a look at the Book of the Prophet Isaiah can enlighten us a bit more about what it means for the Lord to "call one by name." In his writing the great prophet assures us that God has "redeemed" the people He had called His own and will guide and protect them from any "ordeal."[15] Yahweh, as described by the prophet Isaiah, will also bless those who experience pain and trouble in His service as evidenced in one of his servant songs entitled "The Suffering Servant." In this song, which seems to present a foretelling of the sufferings of the Messiah to come, one called by name to be God's servant, although perhaps having suffered greatly, "shall be exalted and lifted up" (*Isaiah* 52:13).[16]

These thoughts from Isaiah can be very consoling to nurses called to care for the sick and suffering for they also suffer with their ill patients. Sometimes I wonder what it is that encourages so many women and men to feel "called by name" to serve the ill and the infirm. When I pose the question, I am always deeply moved by the responses of young nurses who share their thoughts. Such a personal calling was described by 24-year-old pediatric nurse Katie:

> I do feel called by God to be a nurse. From the time I was in high school I wanted to care for sick people; to take care of them when they really are needy. I think God did call me, Katie, by my name because I wanted so much to be a nurse. Nursing just seems to fit me. There are so many opportunities to care for people; opportunities to care for Jesus, really, as He said in the Bible. You know, whenever you do for my little ones, you do for me.

Katie's perception reflects well what it means for those of us who are nurses to be "called by name" to care for the sick. Most nurses whom I have encountered in practice, teaching, or research are very clear about the fact that they would rather do nursing than be engaged in any other profession. They feel "called by name" to care for their more frail and fragile brothers and sisters, and they believe indeed that this personal calling to serve is from the "Lord ... who created" them (*Isaiah* 43:1).

SERVE ONE ANOTHER

Like good stewards of the manifold grace of God, serve one another
with whatever gift each of you has received.

1 Peter 4:10

In Peter's first letter to the dispersed Christian community, he spoke of concepts such as living a holy life, imitating the example of Christ's suffering, and, in chapter 4, becoming "good stewards of God's grace" and serving one another "with whatever gifts" each one had received (4:10). In commenting on chapter 4, verse 10 of Peter's letter, Jerome Neyrey observed that Christians are called to display distinctive virtues, including "constant love, hospitality and generosity." ... Christian duties ... "singled out for special emphasis" included "generous service" to others.[17]

Nursing gives us an incredible opportunity to "serve one another" with love and generosity, using the precious gift of caring for the sick with which we have been blessed by the Lord. There are, of course, a variety of service-oriented vocations in fields such as teaching, social work, child-care and child-protective services, police work, fire-fighting, and many others. A uniqueness of nursing, however, is that we care primarily for those who are in some way in need of support associated with their health or that of loved ones. And we can be confident that the underlying philosophy of our calling was derived from the Gospel message of Jesus who taught us to care for the sick as a way of serving each other.

I love hearing nurses' stories of serving such as that of Pattie who related one of the Lord's maxims from the Sermon on the Mount to a patient care experience. Pattie told about caring for an elderly gentleman who had suffered numerous strokes and had not regained full mobility of one arm and leg. He was feeling very sad and depressed over his physical losses. He was grieving the loss of the health and strength that he once possessed. Pattie reported that she was not always sure if her patient was understanding her, but one day she took his hand and squeezed it and read him a biblical message: "Blessed are they who mourn for they shall be comforted." Pattie added, "I had to repeat this quote several times but I knew that I had struck a chord. Toward the end of our time together [the patient] indicated that he wanted to get involved in his prayer life again. He wanted to get spiritually well even though he knew he could not be physically strong ever again."

Pattie concluded, "It was really great to see this transformation in him and to witness God working through my serving my patient."

Nurses serve in many ways: physical, emotional, and spiritual, sometimes using a combination of all three dimensions of patient care in holistic nursing. Although a patient's physical needs may initially seem to demand a nurse's primary concern and attention, especially in the case of critically ill patients in settings such as the emergency department or intensive care unit, emotional and spiritual needs cannot long be neglected. These latter needs may be powerfully influential in patient healing and even survival, on occasion.

I remember a patient I cared for some years ago, when serving as head nurse of an orthopedic ward in a large Midwest inner-city hospital. Mrs. Kelly, a lovely lady in her late seventies, had been admitted for a fractured hip, an injury incurred by so many older adults. Mrs. Kelly had surgery to repair her hip and seemed initially to be doing very well; she had a good appetite and was a delightfully compliant and cheery patient. Mrs. Kelly's daughter and family visited frequently. One day, however, the patient's daughter told the staff, as she had just admitted to her mother, that this would be their last visit for some time; the family was moving to California. To Mrs. Kelly it seemed like they were moving to another country. She cried quietly after the family left and then did not speak of it again.

Gradually at first and then more precipitously each day, Mrs. Kelly began a downward spiral physically. She no longer seemed to care about ambulating or getting well; she virtually stopped eating, only picking at her food. All the staff nurses were worried about the grieving patient. We tried everything we knew to support and encourage Mrs. Kelly, to lift her spirits. We alerted the orthopedic surgeon who visited on numerous occasions. But several weeks after her family's departure for California, our patient developed a severe case of pneumonia with complications and passed away. The hospital staff were shocked and frustrated. Mrs. Kelly's surgeon commented sadly, "There was nothing we could have done; she didn't die of a broken hip, she died of a broken heart."

Sometimes nurses are not successful, as hard as we may try, to help a patient cope with a stressful life situation. My experience with Mrs. Kelly taught me, graphically and painfully, the importance of a patient's emotional and spiritual needs in regard not only to the healing process but to survival itself.

MAKE A JOYFUL NOISE: THE NURSE AS GOD'S *FLUTE*

Make a joyful noise to the Lord, all the earth; break forth into joyous song and sing praises.

Psalm 98:4

In a poignant meditation entitled "Instruments of God," spiritual writer Joyce Rupp uses the metaphor of "a small wooden flute," a "hollow reed," resting in "the hand of God" to reflect a spiritual posture one may adopt as in serving the Lord and each other.[18] The purpose of one's identifying as "God's flute" is so that he or she may be used as an instrument by which the Lord can make music for the "song starved world."[19]

A similar use of the reed flute as spiritual metaphor for servanthood was identified by British writer Caryll Houselander in her classic work, *The Reed of God.* In the book Houselander describes Mary, the Mother of Jesus, as God's flute or reed "through which the Eternal Love was to be piped as a shepherd's song."[20] Houselander notes, "It is emptiness like the hollow in the reed...which can have only one destiny; to receive the piper's breath and to utter the song that is in his heart."[21] Caryll Houselander goes on to point out that as the material for a flute, a reed must be "cut by a sharp knife, hollowed out" with "stops ... cut in it;" "it must be shaped and pierced before it can utter the shepherd's song."[22] "Thus," Houselander observes, "it is with us; we may be formed by the knife, pared down ... to the minimum of our being"[23] to become God's flute, to be used to sing His melody with our lives.

I find the spiritual metaphor of becoming God's flute most appropriate for the ministry of nursing; the ministry of serving the ill and the infirm, for surely the sick constitute a community of our brothers and sisters who desperately need to be comforted by the melody of God's love. The spirituality of the flute, which can support nursing, is embedded not only in the spiritual literature but in the scriptures as well.

In discussing musical instruments identified in scripture, *Harper's Bible Dictionary* notes that the "flute" or "pipe" was the "principal biblical wind instrument;" the flute could be used on "joyful occasions ... but it was also suitable for mourning."[24] We find the flute referred to in a number of Old Testament passages such as the *First Book of Kings* 1:39–40, which contains a description of the joyful celebration of King Solomon's accession to the throne of Israel: "Then they blew the trumpet, and all the people said, 'Long live King Solomon!' And all the people went up following him, playing on pipes (flutes) and rejoicing with great joy."

The flute is mentioned in the book of Job as being used to express both joy and sorrow. In *Job*, chapter 21, verse 12, Job speaks about how some people live to old age, happily with seemingly no problems; he comments, "They sing to the tambourine and the lyre; and rejoice to the sound of the flute." Later in the book, however, as Job is describing the struggles that have beset his own life, he reports, "My lyre is turned to mourning and my flute to the voice of those who weep" (30:31). And in the final song of the Book of Psalms, *Psalm* 150, in which the psalmist suggests how people should praise the Lord for His "surpassing greatness," we are taught to praise God with "lute and harp" and with "strings and pipe" (verses 3–4). Thus we find Old Testament interpretations of the flute understood as an instrument of joy, sorrow, and praise.

Use of the flute as an instrument of spiritual expression is also found in the New Testament, for example, in Matthew's account of Jesus' visit to the home of Jairus, the Synagogue leader whose daughter the community feared was dead: "When Jesus came to the leader's house and saw the flute players and the crowd making a commotion, he said, 'Go away; for the girl is not dead but sleeping'" (9:23–24). And in a passage in Matthew, chapter 11, Jesus is quoted, in context of praising John the Baptist, as likening the current confused generation to children, calling to each other: "We played the flute for you and you did not dance; we wailed and you did not mourn" (11:17); in this narrative the flute is presented by Jesus as an instrument supportive of joy and celebration in dance. Again, in the New Testament, the flute is presented as an instrument used in a time of sorrow, at the believed death of Jairus' daughter, and as a vehicle for joyful musical expression supportive of dance.

But what does it mean for us, as nurses, to consider ourselves, as suggested by spiritual writers Joyce Rupp and Caryll Houselander, to be God's "flutes." I have pondered this question, related to my own life, both personal and professional. And I have adopted the metaphor of the "flute" to help me understand the meaning of my nursing ministry. Symbolic of this, I keep a small wooden flute, which a friend found for me at a yard sale, on a prayer table in my room next to my Bible. It's a very simple unvarnished reed pipe, battered and worn from use, but I like that about it; even its bruises seem very appropriate to remind me that being God's flute may bring about significant wear and tear, including some distinctive scars.

At this point in my nursing career, writing and teaching are the primary ways in which I can be used as God's flute, as His instrument in ministering to the ill and the infirm. It is the same for many of us who "nurse" in the academic setting. Although we may not immediately see the fruits of our ministry, being God's flute means allowing ourselves to be constantly open to the breath of the Holy Spirit; in this posture our professional activities of research, writing, and teaching are grounded in God's love and centered on proclaiming God's message of compassion in our plans of care for sick brothers and sisters.

For those whose nursing is embedded in roles as managers and administrators, there are myriad opportunities to be used as God's flutes in day-to-day interactions with health care staff. Nurses who take on the heavy burdens that rest on the shoulders of those who supervise others have not only the responsibility but also the blessing of serving as witnesses to God's tenderness, God's understanding, and even God's forgiveness of error or weakness, in interacting with staff over whom they exercise power and authority. To be perceived as a gentle and just and caring administrator or manager by subordinates is one of the greatest accolades that can be awarded to a nurse whose primary role is to supervise others; surely he or she is the lived embodiment of God's covenant with His people.

And finally, the nurse practitioner or the practicing nurse in hospital, clinic, school, home, or physician's office has an exquisite opportunity to serve as God's flute in interaction with his or her patients, especially with those who are most fragile and in need of kindness and understanding. Opportunities for compassionate caregiving abound in emergency departments, critical care units, hospices, hospital wards, and virtually every setting where nurses minister to patients and their families. In this ministry of serving as the Lord's flute, nurses can live out a covenant of caring as described by God the Father in the Old Testament scripture and by the Divine Son Jesus in the New Testament passages.

A SACRED COVENANT

I have made a covenant with my chosen one.

Psalm 89:3

My research with patients and their caregivers over the years has definitively revealed the nurse–patient relationship to be a covenant, to be, in fact, a bonding described earlier as a "sacred covenant."[25-27]

The sacredness of the nurse's caring relationship with a patient derives directly from the sacredness of the nurse's vocation, of his or her call to care for the most vulnerable members of our society: the ill and the infirm.

But what does the word "sacred" mean for us as nurses? How is it that we dare to describe both our calling and our patient relationships as sacred? The concept of sacredness has been associated with such attributes as holiness, closeness to God, spirituality, and religiosity or religious practice. Recognizing someone or something as sacred can make us step back, somewhat in awe of the meaning and power embedded in the adjective. And so it should be with our precious vocation of ministering to the sick, our covenant to care for God's fragile ones.

The sacredness, the holiness, of the nursing vocation of caring for the sick traces its history to the time of Jesus and His first disciples. Jesus not only healed many ill and disabled Himself but He proclaimed the ministry to His followers in such mandates as "Cure the sick … cleanse the lepers, cast out demons" (*Matthew* 10:8). Jesus further supported the importance of nursing the ill with the words, "I was sick and you took care of me … truly, I tell you, just as you did it to one of the least of these who are members of my family, you did it to me" (*Matthew* 25:36, 40).

The true sacredness of the nurse–patient covenant is best exemplified in the real-life experiences of practicing nurses such as that of Andrea, a parish nurse, who was willing to assume a variety of activities to comfort her anxious patient. Andrea told a covenant story in describing her commitment to Mrs. O'Connor: "Mrs. O'Connor is a woman in her seventies who suffers from a multitude of health problems and found herself unable to care for herself; this necessitated her moving to an assisted care facility. Mrs. O'Connor's short-term memory was shot, and although she remembered me (from a previous visit) that was about her only recollection."

Andy reported that Mrs. O'Connor was a "worrier": "I talked to her very simply and was able to minister to her by focusing on the small things she was worrying about. Helping her place calls to her family, helping her tidy her apartment, whatever it might be. I focused on one scripture passage and repeated it each time we met. The passage was *Matthew* 6:33–34: '*But seek first the kingdom of God and his rightousness, and all those things will be given you besides. Do not worry about tomorrow; tomorrow will take care of itself. Sufficient for a day is its own evil.*' "

Andy remained committed to her covenant of caring for Mrs. O'Connor despite her patient's memory loss and worries. She noted that Mrs. O'Connor herself told her on each visit, "I know you are going to tell me not to worry and to let tomorrow take care of itself." Andy added, "That was the only short-term recall that I witnessed (Mrs. O'Connor) accurately repeating over the course of a number of visits."

Andy concluded, "I hope I was able to reach her, and on some level I'm confident that I did. I just hope I was able to bring her a little peace, but then again," Andy added wryly, "I probably should not worry!"

This chapter examined the concept of "sacred covenant" as lived out in the real world of nursing practice, of the nurse–patient relationship. Poignant stories of caring and compassion shared by nurses reflect the "sacredness" of the relationship. The covenantal concepts of "faithfulness" and "unconditional commitment to be of service" are demonstrated repeatedly in the nurses' clinical anecdotes. Those who, as Andy, shared their stories not only described tender experiences of patient care but also validated the "sacredness" of nursing as a holy calling from the perspective of personal satisfaction in caregiving. Nurses felt blessed and gifted in their chosen profession.

Each of the chapter's key concepts support the overall theme of viewing nursing as a "Sacred Covenant." Being called to care for the sick is a "holy calling" as identified by Jesus Himself in His Gospel messages. And as individual followers of the Lord, nurses are "called by name" to "serve one another" in our ministry to the sick. We have the treasured opportunity to be God's "flutes," making a "joyful noise" in our work of healing and caring. Ultimately, all of our caregiving activities combine to form a "Sacred Covenant" that is the blessed vocation of nursing.

A NURSE'S PRAYER OF COVENANT

Thus (God) has shown the mercy promised to our ancestors and remembers His holy covenant.

Luke 1:72

Lord of my life and my heart, I bless You for calling me to a sacred covenant of caring for the sick. Teach me to revere this covenant as a treasured gift as I minister to the ill and the infirm. Let my nursing covenant be graced with Your compassion, with Your tenderness, with Your gentleness, with Your care, and with Your love. Guide my covenantal ministry of caring that it may always reflect the holy vocation to which I have been called. Help me to be worthy. Amen.

2　Ministers of a New Covenant: The Spirituality of Caregiving

Our competence is from God, who has made us competent to be ministers of a new covenant, not of letter but of Spirit.

2 Corinthians 3:5–6

MINISTERS OF A NEW COVENANT

Nurses are called to be ministers of a new covenant:

Nurses are called to minister to the poor in spirit, that they may become rich in the caring;

Nurses are called to minister to those who mourn, that they may find comfort in their sorrow;

Nurses are called to minister to the meek, that they may find strength for the challenges of illness;

Nurses are called to minister to those who hunger and thirst for righteousness, that they may find peace in their suffering;

Nurses are called to minister to
those who are persecuted, that
they may find succor in the
heart of a caregiver.

Bless, Dear Lord, our precious
ministry of nursing.

Are nurses really meant to be "ministers"? I have been exploring that question in my research and writing for the past decade and a half. I believe that this chapter will help answer concerns of those who are in doubt. Because I love hunting through the historical nursing literature for "buried" treasures to support my thoughts, I searched for mention of the concept of ministry in a number of early nursing texts. Our forebears did indeed view nursing as encompassing ministry. I especially like the understanding of registered nurse Jane Hudson, author of *How to Become a Trained Nurse,* published in 1897. Nurse Hudson asserted the following in her introductory chapter entitled, "What it is to be a nurse": "Nurses must be ministers in every sense of the word ... viewed with all the high possibilities involved; no other calling can be greater or nobler than that of the trained nurse."[1]

In Chapter 1, the concept of the nurse–patient relationship, envisioned as a "sacred covenant," drew its spiritual grounding from the Old Testament concept of God's covenant with His people, as articulated by the author of the book of Genesis. In this chapter we look to the New Testament concept of covenant, as described by Saint Paul in his second letter to the Corinthians.

The covenant of the New Testament revolves around the incarnation and redemption accomplished through God's sending of His Divine Son to atone for the weaknesses of humankind. Jesus becomes the advocate for humanity before His Father. Thus when Paul suggests that Christian followers of the Lord may be "ministers of a new covenant," he observes that Christians are "letters of Christ," those who are to go forth to live and preach the Gospel message taught by Jesus, the consummate minister of the new covenant.

Saint Paul explains, further, that he and we may have confidence in undertaking this ministry, not because of our own abilities and talents but only because we have been called by God, and that this is a confidence that comes "through Christ." Paul asserted, "Not that we are competent of ourselves to claim anything as coming from us; our competence is from God, who has made us competent to be ministers of a new covenant, not of letter but of Spirit" (*2 Corinthians* 3:5-6). Biblical scholar Mary Ann Getty points out that Paul's explanation of the ministry of the new covenant was, in part, a response to questions and concerns from the early Corinthian community. Getty notes, "Although no one could conceivably be qualified for this mission (see *2 Corinthians* 2:16), the God who created and who made the covenant written in stone, now recreates and qualifies ministers for the new covenant."[2]

This teaching of Paul is especially important for nurses in our ministry of compassion and caring. I know that I, and I'm sure many other nurses, have at times felt overwhelmed with the immensity of the ministry of caregiving to which we are called. This is especially true in nursing those with devastating life-threatening illnesses for which there is currently no cure. We might sometimes wonder if we are personally prepared to face the suffering our patients experience, much less be able to provide the kind of supportive care to help them cope. It is in situations such as this that we need to summon up the confidence that comes "through Christ" to be His ministers, the confidence that will enable us to move "into deep water" in our caring nurse–patient relationships.

INTO DEEP WATER

When He had finished speaking (Jesus) said to Simon, 'Put out into deep water and let down your nets for a catch.

Luke 5:4

I have to confess that I don't remember a lot of direct quotes from my school of theology faculty members, but a statement from a wonderful Franciscan professor has haunted me for some years now. At the beginning of one of our moral theology classes, he challenged us with the comment, "Jesus is asking you to go out into the "deep water," to stop hanging on to the shore for security." I can't recall the specific words my professor used to elaborate on the challenge but I know that he touched my spirit profoundly. And, ever since that day, when considering a new ministry or even some activity involving my current ministry of writing and teaching, I wonder if I am really willing to go out into the "deep water" where Jesus would have me go or whether I am holding on to the safety of the shoreline with all my might.

Jerome Kodell, commenting on Luke's description of Jesus' call to Simon to "put out into deep water" observed that "Simon is called to obedience based on faith" and adds "It was certainly not reason that provoked this fisherman to cast his nets back into the water at the instigation of this carpenter from the inland hills…. But Simon placed his trust in Jesus."[3] Must we not also do as Simon when called by Jesus in our nursing to enter into "deep water" in our patient interactions?

Going into deep water can be scary, and seemingly irrational, as Kodell points out. I can still vividly recall my first experience of literally entering deep water as a 10-year-old summer camper. I had been attending a girls' camp in the Pennsylvania mountains for a couple of years and one of my favorite activities was swimming. Being small for my age, however, I had been kept in the roped-off "baby" section of the lakefront until I acquired the requisite swimming ability to go into deeper water. I was also forced to wear a despised "red cap" that limited my aquatic activities to water not over my head; this meant simply paddling around the shallow end of the lake rather than actually swimming, which I longed to do.

Finally, during my third summer as a season camper, I was told that I would be allowed to take the test to achieve a treasured "green cap;" this would allow me to swim in a larger deeper area of the lake. I was thrilled. I was also scared to death. The test involved diving off the camp dock into deep water over my head and swimming approximately 50 feet to the shore.

I remember quite clearly standing frozen at the edge of the white-washed dock, my stomach tied in knots, as I gazed down into what seemed like the deepest and darkest water I had ever seen. (It was really only about 15 feet, but for a 10-year-old that seemed like an awfully long way down and, of course, in a freshwater lake you can't see the bottom.) I'm not quite sure what got me moving that day, perhaps it was simply the thought of the lusted-after green cap, but I finally dived into the water, forgetting to hold my breath and coughing and sputtering, paddled furiously. I passed the test, got my treasured green cap, and have loved swimming ever since. The moral of my story is this: Going into "deep water" is frightening but the reward is glorious!

I think that all nurses have had experiences of jumping into "deep water" in their previous lives; these can, I believe, prepare us for nurse-patient situations that may also involve entering into deep water. I had such a nursing experience when, as a young student, I was assigned to care for Vincent, a post-polio patient. Vincent had come to live at our hospital after a year at a rehabilitation facility; he was not able to breathe on his own, being paralyzed from the neck down, as one of the country's last victims of bulbar polio. Vincent brought with him myriad medical technological aids, which most of us had never seen, including a rocking bed, a Monaghan portable respirator, a chest-shell respirator, and even an iron lung for emergencies.

I entered Vincent's room for the first time with a great deal of fear and trepidation. Aside from his medical condition I knew that Vincent was a seminarian, studying for the priesthood. I not only did not know how to care for him physically, but I was not sure how he was handling his extreme state of incapacitation. I wondered how I, a student nurse, could provide the needed physiological and psychological care and support that Vincent needed; I prayed to Our Lady and her Son for help. I knew that I couldn't do it on my own.

As it turned out Vincent became my teacher and my spiritual support. He had learned well, at the rehab center, how to explain to caregivers the intricacies of his machinery and the needs of his paralyzed body. And Vincent's spirit was magnificent to behold. In the several years during which I cared for him, I never heard him complain — not once! He would listen to my worries and concerns but never belabor his own. I knew that Vincent desperately hoped he could regain strength in his arms and hands so that he might one day be able to consecrate bread and wine as a priest at the altar. This was not to be, however, and so he accepted his limitation and thanked God and those who ministered to him with joy and love. All who entered Vincent's room felt blessed to be in his presence; those of us who cared for him were doubly blessed. Vincent became one of my dearest friends and most treasured spiritual mentors. As I suggested earlier, going into "deep water" is frightening but the reward is glorious!

To go back to the original scripture, which was the catalyst for my relating personal "deep water" experiences, what Jesus was really asking by His request to "put out into deep water" was, of course, absolute trust in His will. I'm sure it must have been a challenge for Simon, after a long night of fishing with no catch, to listen to Jesus and "put out into deep water." And yet Simon did it!

And isn't that what the Lord asks of all of His followers, to live the gospel message and trust, even if things are not going the way we might wish. One strategy for understanding the gospel, which some spiritual directors advise, is to place yourself in the particular passage you are reading, to be a bystander observing the interaction of those involved in the story. I'm afraid that if I were to become a "bystander" in Luke's account of the Lord's call to Simon, I might think to myself, "Whoa! Why is this young rabbi, whose trade is carpentry, trying to advise seasoned fishermen when and where they should cast their nets? Don't they know the seas better than he? Why are they trusting his advice?"

This is a scary scenario for me because it makes me wonder if, in fact, I respond like that; if I make decisions about how to live my life based on what I think is best rather than what the Lord is trying to teach me in His gospel message. Placing oneself in the midst of a gospel passage can indeed shed new light on the meaning of the biblical teaching.

THE NURSE AT THE WELL

A Samaritan woman came to draw water and Jesus said to her, 'Give me a drink.'... (Jesus added) If you knew the gift of God, and who it is that is saying to you 'Give me a drink,' you would have asked him, and he would have given you living water... those who drink of the water I will give them will never be thirsty.

John 4:7, 10, 14

I mentioned in the earlier anecdote describing my first nursing foray into deep water that I had sought help from Jesus and His Mother. I prayed for my nursing to be supported by life-giving Divine guidance so that I might not drown in the midst of such deep water. That is what Jesus is teaching us to do in His parable of the "woman at the well."

The Lord, tired from traveling, sat down at a well and asked a Samaritan woman for a drink of water. The woman questioned Jesus as to why he, a Jew, would even speak to her. Jesus explained that if the woman had recognized who he was, "God's gift," she would in turn have asked him for a drink, and the water that he would give, the living water of eternal life, would prevent her from ever being thirsty again. Jesus' offer of living water "symbolically represents God's gift that comes through Jesus—revelation, the Holy Spirit, eternal life;"[4] the evangelist John pictures the water as "life giving, welling up into eternal life."[5]

Nurses throughout the history of our profession have found that "going to the well" in prayer has provided their strength and their sustenance. Florence Nightingale was known as a woman of prayer. In an 1846 letter written to a family member, Florence divulged a moving daily reflection: "I never pray for anything temporal ... but when each morning comes, I kneel down before the rising sun and only say: 'Behold the handmaid of the Lord, give me this day my work to do, no, not my work but Thine.' "[6]

There are many ways in which nurses can "go to the well" in prayer. There is formal communal prayer with one's faith community or personal meditative prayer prayed alone either in church or simply walking in a park or resting in one's home. One way of praying that some nurses find helpful is to pray with scripture. A more formalized way of praying with scripture is called *Lectio Divina* or Divine Reading. In this method one chooses a meaningful biblical passage and reads it very slowly and meditatively. When a particular word, phrase, or sentence touches the spirit, it is suggested that the reading be stopped and that part of the scripture now guide one's prayer. There are myriad biblical passages and anecdotes related to illness and healing that might be meaningful sources of prayer for nurses.

Rachel, a parish nurse, related a personal experience of using scripture in "going to the well" in her caring for Mrs. Moran, a woman suffering from a debilitating neurological illness. Rachel described the fact that she had numerous interactions with the patient but was not really sure if she "had helped the woman" in coping with her illness or in her faith. Rachel admitted that when she returned home after one of her visits with Mrs. Moran, she was very discouraged. "But," she added, "I got home that day and (read the passage from 2 Corinthians 1: 3–4): *'Blessed be the God and Father of our Lord Jesus Christ, the Father of compassion and God of all encouragement, who encourages us in our every affliction, so that we may be able to encourage those who are in any affliction with the encouragement with which we ourselves are encouraged by God.'"*

Rachel concluded, "This passage really struck me, and it has kind of become my mantra in getting ready to go out and minister to my patients. It gives me strength, and reminds me that God comforted me, and that I am able to use that same peace to comfort others; this is a real source of prayer for me."

TO BRING GOOD NEWS

The Spirit of the Lord is upon me, because he has anointed me to bring good news.

Luke 4:17

I wondered, at first, if "to bring good news" was an appropriate message for nurses caring for those who are ill. At times, of course, we are able to bring good medical news to our patients or their families. It is a joy, and a source of nursing satisfaction, when we can share the good news of things such as a positive response to therapy, satisfactory lab test results, or the presence of good vital signs. Nurses must also sometimes be the bearers of not so good news. We may have to inform a patient of unexpected health-related occurrences such as a dangerous rise in blood pressure, an abnormal temperature, or a delay in anticipated hospital discharge.

In the context of whatever medical or nursing information we have to relay to patients or families, however, nurses can, with our concern and our caring and our commitment, bring the "good news" of the Gospel message of Jesus. We can be used, as noted in the previous chapter, as the hands and the feet and the eyes of Christ in ministering to our suffering patients. We can relate whatever news we must to patients and families with gentleness and empathy. And we can learn how to do this from the biblically reported life of Jesus.

The evangelist Luke recorded Jesus' announcement that he had been anointed by the Spirit to "bring good news;" Jesus is "the spirit-bearer foretold by Isaiah (*Isaiah* 11:2), the Prophet and Messiah who will usher in a new age of freedom and divine favor."[7] In the same scripture passage, Jesus is also quoted as proclaiming that he has been sent to bring that "good news" to groups of persons who are disabled or in some way marginalized from society: those who are being held captive by some condition, those whose sight has been compromised, and those oppressed by the weight of heavy burdens.

All nurses are called, in their ministry of caring, to "proclaim the good news" as described in Luke's Gospel: "to proclaim good news to the poor...to proclaim release to captives and recovery of sight to the blind, to let the oppressed go free" (4:18). In our work of ministering to the sick we proclaim the good news of our caring to the "poor" each day. For some, our nursing may be with patients who are materially poor and marginalized from the larger society; for other nurses their patients' illness, including the loss of physical or cognitive abilities, constitute a poverty of health equally as grave as material poverty.

Regardless of the particular kind of poverty experienced by those for whom we care, nurses have a blessed opportunity to bring the good news of God's love and tender concern for all of His people, especially for those suffering loss. As Jesus has told us repeatedly, it was for the poor and the needy that He came, for the ill and the infirm. As the Divine Physician reminded the Pharisees, "Those who are well have no need of a physician, but those who are sick" (*Matthew* 9:12). Jesus added, "Go and learn what this means, I desire mercy not sacrifice" (9:13). We, as nurses, sharing and living the good news of Jesus' gospel have the vocation of mercy in our daily duties of ministering to the needs of our poor sick patients and their families.

And in this ministry of mercy, of proclaiming the "good news," nurses also have the graced opportunity of modeling Jesus' mandate in assisting captives to be released, the blind to recover their sight, and the oppressed to go free. We can help those persons captive and oppressed by their illness and infirmities to know and experience the freedom and relief from burden that comes through faith in Jesus and hope for wellness and joy in eternal life, for which we have been created. We can also assist the sick, blinded to God's love, to allow the "scales to fall from their eyes" and "see" and understand the Father's love and tenderness in the midst of their pain and suffering.

Hospital Chaplain Cornelius van der Poel observed, "Concerns for the sick and the well-being of all people are the clearest examples of ministry in the life of Jesus. They manifest his compassion for the afflicted."[8] How blessed we nurses are to be able to follow the Lord Jesus' compassion in bringing "good news" to the sick, especially those who sit in darkness and the shadow of death.

I witnessed Barbara, a parish nurse, lovingly bringing "good news" to a nursing home resident when accompanying her on a Sunday afternoon visit. The patient, Mrs. Flatley, was a 49-year-old Roman Catholic who was in the nursing home because of a diagnosis of ovarian cancer with metastasis; she had very little family to support or care for her. The nursing home was a nonsectarian care facility with no religious symbols anywhere in evidence. On a previous meeting Mrs. Flatley had told her parish nurse that she would love to have a small statue of the Sacred Heart. On our visit Barbara brought the patient not only a statue of the Sacred Heart but one of Our Lady and a small rosary. Mrs. Flatley began to cry she was so happy. She kissed the statues and held them close to her heart. Then she asked us to put them on her table so that she could see them first thing every morning when she awoke. She also kissed the Crucifix on her rosary and said it was "just exactly" the kind of rosary she loved. We spoke to Mrs. Flatley about her faith, and she told us how much our visit meant to her. She admitted to sadness over an earlier phone call from her son, for whom she had been waiting all day; he told her that he was "running late" and would not be able to visit.

Mrs. Flatley added, "It made the day a little bit down but now it's back up in such a special way because God sent you to me."

WHERE TWO OR THREE ARE GATHERED

For where two or three are gathered in my name, I am there among them.

                                                              Matthew 18:20

Jesus told us that where even two or three of His followers were gathered "in His name" He would be in their midst. This is a very real and a very powerful message. Biblical scholars note that Jesus was promising that when the "community," which may be as few as two people, come together in prayer, "the prayer will be accepted by God as binding,"[9] and that the "cohesive center of this praying community is ultimately the presence of Jesus."[10]

Several ways in which Christian nurses can bring the "good news" of the gospel are through prayer, scripture reading, or even listening and engaging in spiritual discussions with our patients. In these blessed interactions where nurse and patient come together in Jesus' name, the Lord indeed is present lovingly guiding, supporting, and inspiring His disciples to comprehend and live His proclamation of the coming of the Kingdom.

Over the years I have heard many beautiful stories of what I have labeled "nursing liturgies."[11] A nursing anecdote that poignantly reflects a prayerful sharing in Jesus' name was that related by Annie, a clinic nurse: "We had sent one of our patients from the Cardiology Clinic to the Emergency Department because he was having a heart attack. After he was transported he immediately underwent coronary artery bypass graft surgery to alleviate the blocked arteries. I went to visit him a couple of days later. He was a relatively young man, only in his forties, and he was very scared about what this meant. He was petrified about what had happened, about the fact that he could have died and left his children without a father."

Annie continued, "When I arrived at his room he was absolutely panicked. I did not know what religious affiliation he was but I saw no other way to help him than to sit down right there and pray with and for him. I held his hand and began to pray. I did most of the talking, and just asked the Lord to ease his pains and his anxieties, to show him the way, to help him recuperate, to bless him and his family, and for the patient to develop a deeper relationship with God and His power in his life."

Annie added, "I felt an energy move through me to him, something I had never felt before in the times I've prayed with people. It was intense and moving, and the instant transformation in the patient was indescribable. He seemed at peace; his pulse rate and blood pressure dropped. He told me that he had been raised Catholic but had not been to church for years. He told me that my prayer was absolutely beautiful and a turning point for him. He said that he wanted to pray again, and that if the Lord could help him through this, he wanted to come back to the Church."

Annie concluded, "He started praying that day. Over the next few weeks I saw the most amazing changes in this man. He relied on the Lord to help him get well, to provide for him and his family. He returned to church and the following Easter his wife and children were baptized."

An important point to remember about Annie's story is that she had no idea of her patient's religious affiliation or background, and this nursing opportunity to call on the Lord "where two or three are gathered" would not have occurred if Annie had not taken the risk to pray, the risk to try the one ministry she thought might help her frightened, anxious, post-op patient.

YOU TOOK CARE OF ME

I was sick and you took care of me.... Truly I tell you, just as you did it to one of the least of these who are members of my family, you did it to me.

Matthew 25:36, 40

To me this teaching of Jesus is the heart of the nursing vocation. How incredibly gifted we are, as nurses, to be able to care for Jesus. We don't consider this very often, I'm sure, in our day-to-day nursing activities. Perhaps it would just be too overwhelming if we did. But imagine how blessed we would feel if we walked into a patient room and discovered Jesus, in his human form, awaiting our caring. It's almost too much to absorb. But just listen again to Our Lord's own words: *"I was hungry and you gave me food, I was thirsty and you gave me drink, a stranger and you welcomed me, naked and you clothed me, ill and you cared for me"* (*Matthew* 25:35–36). Jesus identifies Himself "with the hungry, the stranger, the poor, the sick and the oppressed;"[12] thus "by serving (them) we serve Christ."[13]

Peggy, a geriatric nurse, described the importance of Jesus' mandate that in caring for the least of His brothers and sisters we also care for Him; this is especially important in those times when a nurse is physically, emotionally, or spiritually fatigued. Peggy admitted, "I have found that nursing can sometimes be draining for me as a caregiver. All too often the people that I work with are so very drained physically or emotionally that sometimes I too become weary and feel as though I am getting nowhere, or I cannot reach a particular person. One such person was Martha, who was terminal and who was very angry and depressed when I first began to care for her." Peggy described one interaction with Martha as a "battle" (Martha was very depressed and believed that God did not care about her): "It was a brutal hour or so, and I left feeling pretty deflated. I spent the next days praying, reflecting and journaling about the encounter. I was bound and determined that I was going to win, get through to her and emerge victorious. I had my ammunition ready and I arrived to see her the next time to learn that she had died from multi-system failure."

Peggy continued, "I returned to my apartment (that evening) feeling pretty dejected; I felt that I had let Martha down. I know that death is a part of life but I felt just drained."

Peggy concluded her story by observing that she believed she had not really had the chance to "care" for Martha and sought an answer in the bible. A familiar scripture passage that gave her comfort was from *John* 16:33: "In the world you will have trouble, but take courage for I (Jesus) have conquered the world."

Peggy's story provides an important reminder that although a nurse's caring may not always seem to have borne fruit in terms of a patient response, the desire and effort to care are in themselves symbols of following of Jesus' mandate to "take care of the sick." Jesus didn't tell us that we had to always excel in everything we did. He only taught that we try to live His gospel message to the best of our abilities, to serve our brothers and sisters with the gifts each one of us have been given (1 *Peter* 4:10).

This chapter presents a response to the question of whether nurses are truly called to be "ministers," to be ministers of God's "new covenant" as explained in the Gospel Message of Jesus. Moving anecdotes reflect nurses' tender ministries carried out in their day-to-day activities of caregiving. Nurses are often asked to step out in faith in their nursing ministries; they are called to go into "deep water" where they may at times feel in "over their heads" and to trust in the Lord. Nurses are asked, in that spirit of trust, to go to the "well" of life-giving water that they may be spiritually prepared to bring "good news" to those for whom they care. Nurses are called to share faith with their patients so that trusting together, Jesus will be in their midst. And finally, in the most blessed vocation of all, nurses are asked to minister to Jesus Himself, for in caring for the least of His brothers, they indeed care for Him.

A NURSE'S PRAYER FOR COURAGE IN MINISTRY

Therefore, since it is by God's mercy that we are engaged in this ministry, we do not lose heart.

2 Corinthians 4:1

Dear Lord Jesus, bless my ministry of nursing that I might never "lose heart" as I care for my frail brothers and sisters, and thus for You, my Lord and my God. Guide my nursing ministry that it may be blessed by Your love and Your understanding and Your gentleness. Let me never forget the gift and the grace and the blessing of being called to minister to the sick in Your name. Help me, dear Lord, to minister to my patients with the Father's care, with the Spirit's wisdom, and with Your passionate commitment and courage. Amen.

3 🕯 Varieties of Gifts: A Tradition of Service

There are varieties of Gifts but the same Spirit.... Varieties of services but the same Lord...it is the same God who activates all of them in everyone.

1 Corinthians 12:4

Like good stewards of the manifold grace of God, serve one another with whatever gift each of you has received.

1 Peter 4:10

A TRADITION OF SERVICE

*Nurses are graced with the gift of
Servanthood; nurses are blessed
to inherit a tradition of service;
nurses are gifted with the
call to serve as Jesus'
disciples.*

*Nurses are gifted to serve with love
those who are lonely and
abandoned.*

*Nurses are gifted to serve with tenderness
those who are broken in body or
in spirit.*

*Nurses are gifted to serve with courage
those who are anxious or
afraid.*

Nurses are gifted to serve with compassion
   those who are sorrowful and
      suffering.

Nurses are gifted to serve with strength
   those who are fragile and
      weak.

Nurses are gifted to follow in the
   footsteps of the Divine Servant
      of all humanity.
Lord Jesus, Bless our gift
   of servanthood.

Saints Paul's and Peter's teachings on the variety of gifts possessed by different individuals and on using those gifts in the service of others are especially relevant for nurses. Our profession is, today, highly specialized. Even young student nurses begin early on expressing thoughts about whether they want to be pediatric nurses, intensive care unit nurses, emergency department nurses, and so forth. Admittedly, the more exciting specialties usually win out; geriatric nursing is not generally high on the list. The nursing students do, however, realize that they each have unique gifts that make them better suited to serving the sick in a particular health care arena.

Of course, first specialty choices are not always life-career choices in nursing. Sometimes after years of ministering in a hospital-based medical or surgical unit, a nurse will feel called to a specialized setting such as that provided in hospice care. The nurse may recognize over time that his or her gifts, developed and enhanced through many patient care interactions, may now be better used in ministry to those facing the end of life.

The important thing about using our nursing gifts is, as noted by Biblical scholar Mary Ann Getty in her commentary on the First Corinthians scripture, "All gifts with which the community is richly endowed must be valued in proportion to their role in building up the body."[1] The vast multitude of nurses practicing, managing, researching, and teaching in our contemporary health care system use their myriad talents and skills to "build up the body" of professional nursing. The body of nursing knowledge and nursing practice is continually growing and developing through the creative sharing of the gifts of nurses committed to a unique and compassionate ministry of caring.

The variety of gifts nurses have been given is immense; this is the beauty and the joy of God's covenantal love for those who care for His sick. All we need do is be open and ask for His support and His guidance and He will bless us 100-fold in our ministry to those in need.

A TRADITION OF SERVICE

Whoever wishes to be great among you must be your servant, and whoever wishes to be first among you must be your slave; just as the Son of Man came not to be served but to serve.

Matthew 20:26–27

Commenting on these words from the gospel of Matthew, scripture scholar Donald Senior points out that, "True greatness in the community of Jesus is not to be determined by rank or by the flex of power. Greatness is determined by how much one is willing to give in the service of others. This is the kind of love that animated Jesus, the Son of Man, who came to serve and to give His life as a ransom for many."[2] "Christ is the enduring model for servanthood ... the form of Christ's servanthood includes self-emptying, identification with the needy, and self-giving."[3] This is the servanthood that the Lord asks of His nurses who care for the sick.

The varieties of gifts with which God has blessed His nurses have been exquisitely evident in our historical tradition of service to the ill and infirm. From the early centuries of the Christian era, when followers of Jesus cared for sick members of their communities, to the present day, nurses have served their more fragile brothers and sisters with whatever talents and abilities God has blessed them. Our foundress, Florence Nightingale, envisioned nursing the sick as a ministry of service, a tradition to be handed down to her followers in a blessed vocation to be cherished and treasured.

Florence revealed her personal image of nursing as a spiritual service in a letter written in 1846 in which she reported asking the Lord, "Give me this day my work to do, no not my work but Thine!"[4] Miss Nightingale's perception of the spiritual ministry of nursing was also demonstrated in the admonition included in her classic 1859 *Notes on Nursing,* "Every nurse...must have a respect for her own calling because God's precious gift of life is often literally placed in her hands"[5] as well as in the oft-cited quote from her unpublished writings, "Nursing is an art, and if it is to be made an art, it requires as exclusive a devotion, as hard a preparation, as any painter's or sculptor's work. For what is having to do with dead canvas or cold marble compared with having to do with the living body, the temple of God's spirit."[6]

Following the lead of their founder, Florence Nightingale, other early nurse scholars also described nursing as having a tradition of service. Isabel Hampton Robb, writing in 1912, observed, "The nurse's work is a ministry; it should represent a consecrated service, performed in the spirit of Christ, who made Himself of no account but went about doing good."[7] Robb added, "The woman who fails to bring this spirit into her nursing misses the pearl of greatest value that is to be found in it."[8]

Author of a classic nursing textbook of the early 20th century, *Textbook of the Principles and Practice of Nursing*, educator Bertha Harmer asserted, "Nursing is rooted in the needs of humanity and is founded on the ideal of service. Its object is not only to cure the sick and heal the wounded but ... to minister to all those who are helpless or handicapped ... the final test, as portrayed in the last Day of Judgment, is ... did ye visit the sick, the poor, the hungry? Nursing includes all of this."[9]

A young nurse, Susan, described a caring experience that exemplifies the teaching of Bertha Harmer that the object of our nursing is not just "to cure the sick and heal the wounded" but to reach out and minister to all those who are helpless or in need. Susan described her interactions with Anna, "a vibrant lady in her late sixties" who was alone and homebound because of her medical conditions and depressed about her illnesses. Anna is "a brittle diabetic who must be monitored closely; she also suffers from neuropathy in her feet and hands." Anna was described as having a "feisty personality" that "might have made her fun to be around as a younger woman;" however, at present Susan admitted, "Her ways wore me down at times and I needed to maintain my own sanity in caring for her!"

Susan stated that she often prayed before entering Anna's room and reflected on *Hebrews* 4:15–16: *"For we do not have a high priest who is unable to sympathize with our weaknesses, but one who has similarly been tested in every way, yet without sin. So let us confidently approach the throne of grace to receive mercy and to find grace for timely help."* Susan added, "I knew that it was God's help and grace and grace alone that would allow me to help Anna and to bring her the peace of the God who loved her so very much."

Susan concluded her anecdote, "I know God used me and is working great things in (Anna's) heart!"

As I read Susan's account of her compassionate care for Anna, it strikes me that although nursing has become much more complex technologically than in the days of our forebears of the late 19th and early 20th centuries, our tradition of service, our tradition of caring, is indeed alive and well as we begin the third millennium. Nurses of the 21st century may be better educated in terms of patients' physiological, psychosocial, and even spiritual needs than those of earlier eras. We may speak in more sophisticated and scholarly language. We may look different from our earlier role models; for some time now crisply starched nursing caps and white uniforms have been passé. But our hearts remain, as first envisioned by Florence Nightingale, focused on the fact that "God's gift of life" is often literally "placed in (our) hands." The heart of a nurse in the 21st century is no different from the heart of a nurse in the 19th century; both are gifted with the blessing of being called to care for the ill and the infirm. This is the true treasure of the "tradition of service" that graces the vocation and profession of nursing.

LOVE ONE ANOTHER

> *I give you a new commandment, that you love one another. Just as I have loved you, you also should love one another. By this everyone will know that you are my disciples, if you have love for one another.*

John 13:34–35

I've often wondered why Jesus said that he was giving us a "new" commandment to love, because the concept of God's love for us as well as our love for Him and for our neighbor seemed to also be central to Old Testament teaching. To cite just a few examples: *Who is like you, O Lord...in your steadfast love you led the people whom you redeemed"* (*Exodus* 15:11, 13); "*You shall love the Lord your God with all your heart, and with all your soul, and with all your might*" (*Deuteronomy* 6:5); "*You shall love your neighbor as yourself*" (*Leviticus* 19:18).

A commentary on the *Gospel of John* addresses the issue of the "new" commandment with the explanation, "The Torah commanded *human* love for ourselves and our neighbor (*Leviticus* 19:18). Jesus commands *divine* love for one another that is modeled on His own acts of charity and generosity (*1 John* 3:16–18). This supernatural love comes not from us but from the Spirit (*Romans* 5:5)."[10] In the words of Neal Flanagan, "It is a *new* commandment because this mutual love must be modeled on something new — on the love that Jesus shows for His disciples. Mutual love must be the sign, the indispensable sign, of their discipleship."[11]

Sharon, a geriatric nurse caring for an ALS (amyotrophic lateral sclerosis) patient residing in a nursing home spoke about caring for her patient as "we ourselves would like to be cared for":

> Michael was generally depressed and angry about his condition and it wasn't until our fourth interaction that I felt that I

really had a breakthrough with him. He said that he wanted to talk about God and had some questions for me. I offered to share some of my faith journey with him and he was interested to hear it. I do not generally talk to patients about my own struggles, but in this case I could see that the man needed something to believe in a tangible witness to the graces and goodness of the Lord. I shared only enough with him so that he could see that I had not always loved God as I should. I was flawed and had needed to overcome my own struggle with a chronic illness.

Sharon continued, "Of course I had to concede to him that he was certainly more drastically physically affected with his illness than I had ever been but that did not mean that God loved him any less. I think hearing about my pain helped him seeing humanity and it gave him some relief. He saw me as a Christian trying to find a way to help him as my fellowman."

Sharon asserted that she believed her attempt to "love another" in this case resulted in her being able to see the patient's "callused heart melt in front of me." After reading the 23rd Psalm together, Michael responded that he wanted to meet with the nursing home chaplain because he stated, "I know that I don't have a lot of time left, and I'm ready to be drawn out from beside the still waters where he has protected me, and rejoice in his glory."

Sometimes patients need only our listening hearts and minds as they verbalize anxieties related to their heavy burdens of illness or disability. At other times a brief sharing of a nurse's own problems can be consoling to a patient in letting the person know that the nurse understands something of the patient's pain and suffering, as in Sharon's interaction with Michael.

When I began a large study of persons living with HIV infections and AIDS, conducted during the early days of the pandemic, some of my nurse team members reported that study participants asked if they would share a little about themselves at first meetings; they wondered if this was appropriate. We asked our psychiatrist consultant for advice. His response was that some minimal sharing of our own experiences was appropriate because we were asking to enter the lives of these very ill patients. This kind of introduction to our patients went a long way in achieving a sense of rapport and helping them to realize they were cared for as persons by the nursing research team. It also helped study participants feel more confident that we were indeed there to take on a part of their burden during our interviews.

BEAR ONE ANOTHER'S BURDENS

Bear one another's burdens, and in that way you will fulfill the law of Christ.

Galatians 6:2

All of Paul's letters to the new communities of Christians with whom he communicated included words of caring, support, encouragement, and teaching. In the above passage of Paul's letter to the Galatians, the apostle was both encouraging and supporting the importance of community, of sharing sorrows and problems as well as joys and successes with each other as members of the Christian family. Saint Paul, who was the most human of men, knew that it was not easy to take on the burdens of others, especially when we already have enough of our own to bear. Thus, he highlighted this point in his teaching, urging the new Galatian Christians "to fulfill the law of Christ by gently helping one another bear any problem that may occur."[12]

Nurses are often called on to "bear the burdens" of their patients. This call is not to undertake a physical burden but rather a psychological, emotional, or spiritual burden that a patient is carrying. How often have we spent time and energy, sometimes time and energy that seemed in short supply on a particular day, listening to the worries and concerns of our anxious patients? Hopefully, our listening and caring was able to, in some measure, alleviate the stress of a patient's burden.

Kelly, a parish nurse, told me a wonderful story of a nurse seeking to "bear (another's) burden." Kelly was assisting at a blood pressure screening activity at her church; she described the caring she observed on the part of one of her colleagues, Chris: "In the middle of the crowd of parishioners there was a man who just seemed despondent; this is extremely uncommon for this group. When it came time for the noticeably quiet and sad man to have his blood pressure checked, Chris sat down and began the process. His reading was too high, particularly above average for him. Chris began to ask him, genuinely concerned, if anything in his life had changed since the last blood pressure reading or if everything was alright. He responded with an unanimated 'Yeah' and began to get up."

Chris immediately asked if he would like to chat for a few minutes about whatever was going on, just so that maybe she could share his burden with him." Kelly continued, "I watched this interaction and to this day I can still see the man's face after Chris asked that. He immediately welled up, and looked at Chris and began to cry softly and some color returned to his pale face. It seemed as though life had been infused back into the man by one simple question. You could tell that he had a deep appreciation for her willingness to listen, to share his burden."

Kelly concluded, "He and Christine spoke for a long time. As it turned out, the man had lost his wife to natural causes about a month prior and his son to suicide about 2 weeks ago. He said that he just felt lost, like he was floundering. He admitted that so many people had asked if he was alright, but after he responded 'no' they seemed to brush him off and just say 'so sorry'. Chris," Kelly added, "was the first person who had taken the time and who cared enough to ask the follow-up question of this stranger."

Finally, Kelly reported, "Chris listened to him, comforted him, and referred him to a local support group where he could find other people who had had to live through tragedies in their lives. What Christine did seems natural for any nurse, I guess, so full of common sense, but it was her taking the time to listen, when so many others would not, that made all the difference for this man and helped him back onto the road of healing."

It's important to point out here that it is not easy to bear "another's burdens," even if this is only done emotionally through listening and verbally supporting a suffering person. When we try to truly empathize with another's pain, we emotionally take at least a part of that pain on our own shoulders and heart. Following nursing research interviews and hospital chaplaincy counseling sessions with seriously ill persons or their family members, I have come away both emotionally and physically drained. There are many stress-reducing techniques suggested for such work, such as walking or running, listening to music, and spending time with friends. All these activities are positive and helpful, but I found that my greatest source of energy and consolation in the work came through prayer and meditation, through seeking the "strength that God supplies."

THE STRENGTH THAT GOD SUPPLIES

Whoever serves must do so with the strength that God supplies, so that God may be glorified in all things through Jesus Christ.

1 Peter 4:11

There are times when we, as nurses, must undertake tasks for which we feel totally unprepared in our ministry of serving the ill and infirm. Because we generally have the medical–technological skills needed for a nursing assignment, such instances generally involve the psychosocial-spiritual realm. It is especially on those occasions that we need to reach out for God's strength.

I remember an experience some years ago when the brother of a critically ill patient in the intensive care unit asked me if I would pray for his sibling. The well brother told me that he himself was not very spiritual but that his brother was and that he knew the prayer would be meaningful to him. This occurred before my doing a hospital chaplaincy program; I was not sure what words I might use that would be comforting to a brother who was not "into," as he put it, religion or spirituality or to his very ill sibling who was. I approached the task by breathing a silent prayer, asking the Lord to give me His words that they might bring some comfort and healing to this suffering pair. In my vulnerability, my insecurity with this request, I desperately needed the strength that only God can supply. And He did! For my simple prayer brought comfort to the brothers.

Pondering this experience reminds me that to receive God's strength so that "God may be glorified in all things," we must have an empty space in our hearts that He alone can fill. If our spirits have become so crowded with perceptions of our own abilities and strengths, there will be no room to receive the blessed gifts that the Lord is waiting to shower on us if only we are open to His love.

It must be admitted, however, that ridding our hearts of excessive material desires and longings to be present to God's love is no easy task. For often such attractions and yearnings are deeply rooted in the very core of our being; they are not easily extracted. And rooted things must be removed whole and entire, lest they simply appear cut back for a time, only to emerge stronger than ever, as new rootlets grow and expand throughout the ground in which they had been planted.

I learned about the difficulty as well as the importance of removing "rooted" things, whole and entire, during an experience of attempting to help Sister Miriam, a religious woman with whom I was living at the time, clear a backyard urban "jungle" of bamboo. For those who are not familiar with bamboo, it is an aggressively growing tropical plant that, once gaining a foothold in fertile soil, spreads like the proverbial wildfire. Plants can grow several inches each day.

The bamboo was literally taking over an area behind our house and needed to be removed to make room for new grass and plants. I, with my nurse academician's soft hands and lack of even a smattering of horticultural knowledge, was ready to just chop off the tops of the bamboo plants, make the yard look better and be done with it! — until Sister Miriam handed me some gloves and a shovel and said, "Start digging! You have to get the roots!" I smiled weakly and begin to dig, perhaps a bit less than enthusiastically, thinking, "This is an impossible task; these roots must go halfway across the country!" Within a few minutes, however, Sister Miriam had put me to shame, showing me how she had exposed a bamboo root with many small rootlets and was now able to pull out the entire plant, leaving no vestiges of the problem shoot to reinstate itself in our yard.

Sister Miriam also carefully showed me how the roots of the plant had branched out in a number of different directions, embedding themselves in many areas of the ground around the original bamboo shoot. The example of the bamboo plant struck me as a spiritual metaphor for explaining the importance of fully "rooting" out frivolous material attractions or enticements that might distract our hearts from seeking the fullness of God's love. Such root extraction cannot be done halfheartedly and without a lot of hard work, as I had wanted to do initially; absolute commitment to completing the task is the only way to succeed.

My experience of working in the bamboo also reminded me of a passage from the beautiful work, *Hinds' Feet on High Places,* an allegory portraying the spiritual journey that each of us must take in our walk with the Lord. Author Hannah Hurnard observes that the only way to reach the "high places" of union with Christ is by "a continually repeated laying down of our own will and acceptance of His."[13] To accomplish this, Hurnard includes, as a central dimension of the allegorical journey, the desire to remove the natural preference for human comfort and satisfaction, rooted in each individual heart; it is suggested that this desire be given up as a "burnt offering" to be fully open to the Divine love of Jesus, the Good Shepherd.

In the end, Hannah Hurnard's protagonist, "Much Afraid," realizes that, of herself, she is not strong enough to remove the deeply rooted human desire: "She knew with a pang, almost of despair, that the roots had wound and twined and thrust themselves into every part of her being. Though she put forth all her remaining strength in the most desperate effort to wrench them out, not a single rootlet stirred."[14] Thus "Much Afraid" begged the Lord, imaged as the "priest of the altar," to remove the roots for her: "The priest put forth a hand of steel, right into her heart. There was a sound of rending and tearing, and the human love, with all its myriad rootlets and fibers, came forth. He held it for a moment and then said: 'Yes, it was ripe for removal, the time had come. There is not a rootlet torn or missing.' "[15]

Many of us, and I place myself at the top of the list, like "Much Afraid," may not have the spiritual strength to "wrench out" from our hearts deeply rooted human desires for untoward material comfort and satisfaction. If, however, we also call upon the Lord, the "priest of the altar," he will never fail to supply the strength for the effort, so that as taught in the First Letter of Saint Peter, *"God may be glorified in all things through Jesus Christ."*

COMMIT YOUR WORK TO THE LORD

Commit your work to the Lord and your plans will be established.
The Lord has made everything for its purpose.

Proverbs 16:3–4

The book of Proverbs contains a variety of maxims that promote "reverence, awe, and respect for the almighty God, who is the creator of heaven and earth" .... Proverbs are not theoretical statements; rather they are affirmations of practical wisdom that help a person to live at peace with himself, with God and with his fellow man."[16] The proverbs "reveal sound psychology and accurate observation of life. They demonstrate the outworking of wisdom and folly in the practical business of living."[17]

The proverb cited above, which advises that if we commit our work to the Lord our plans will be successful, is one of the most basic. This is also a great proverb for nurses to embrace. Nursing is about commitment, commitment of our work to the Lord.

The junior nursing students at the university where I teach recently had their "Commitment to Nursing" ceremony. This is a very solemn ritual, conducted in a church, in which the students through prayer and through extending their hands for a blessing and anointing with holy oil make their commitment to the profession of nursing. The ceremony is undertaken before the initiation of major clinical experiences in which the new nurses will truly begin to experience the meaning of their commitment to caring for the sick. In the course of the ritual, the students do indeed commit their work to the Lord and pray that their journey in nursing education will be blessed and fruitful.

Cindy, a geriatric nurse, reported the fruitfulness of committing her nursing to the Lord in describing an interaction with a patient with whom she had initially been unable to communicate for some time. Katherine was a 72-year-old Christian woman plagued with an acoustic neuroma and severe rheumatoid arthritis; she could only walk limited distances with help, was deaf in one ear, and had very limited vision. Cindy explained, "Katherine lamented about her ailments and the possibility of death, death more imminently than she would like. I quoted to her 1 John 5:11–13: 'God gave us eternal life and this life is in his son ... you have eternal life, you who believe in the name of the Son of God. And we have confidence in him, that if we ask anything according to his will, he hears us!' Cindy continued, "This woman in front of me had such joy on her face that I think God could have called her home right then and she would have been completely okay with that decision. We spent the rest of our time, during all of our remaining visits, talking about what a gift the promise of eternal life is."

Cindy admitted, at the end of her story, "It comforts me to know that God really is in control of these patient interactions, that my nursing is committed to Him, but I have to remember at the same time that I have to surrender the fact that I am not totally in control." Cindy concluded, "The visits with Katherine helped us both, I think, and really allowed me to become more aware of God's love for us and the fact that He has a Divine Plan, so much greater than anything we could imagine."

Throughout this chapter one finds nursing's tradition of service reflected not only in the words of commitment and dedication articulated by our earliest nurse forebears, but also in the clinical anecdotes reported by contemporary nurses such as Cindy and others cited in the preceding pages. From early on nurses have embraced such concepts as service, love, sharing (listening), praying (leaning on God's strength), and commitment to caring for the sick. These values, exquisitely reflected by nurses, are ancient (a tradition of service) and current (nursing commitment ceremonies). These values are the gift and the blessing of nursing.

A NURSE'S PRAYER OF SERVANTHOOD

The Son of Man came not to be served but to serve.

Mark 10:45

O God, who graced our profession of nursing with the precious tradition of servanthood. Teach me to serve. Bless my hands and my heart with Your tenderness and Your love as I seek to serve those who are lonely, those who are afraid, those who are sorrowful, and those who are broken in body or in spirit. Help me to become a true disciple of Your Divine Son who came not to be served but to serve. Let me always treasure the gift of my servanthood, knowing that in caring for ill brothers and sisters I also serve you, my Lord and my God. Amen.

4 Clothed With Compassion: Entering Sacred Spaces

As God's chosen ones, holy and beloved, clothe yourselves with
compassion, kindness, humility, meekness and patience.

Colossians 3:12

CLOTHED WITH COMPASSION

Dear Lord Jesus,
You who had compassion
for all humanity,
Teach Your nurses
the spirituality of
compassionate caring.

Teach us compassion for the frightened child,
tearfully begging to return to home
and family;

Teach us compassion for the stressed preop
patient, anxiously anticipating the
outcome of surgery;

Teach us compassion for the frail elder,
fearfully pondering an uncertain
future;

Teach us compassion for the terminally ill
person, solemnly awaiting the final
exit;

Teach us compassion for the worried family
member, desperately hoping for
a word of reassurance;

Teach us, O Lord, to be nurses
clothed in compassion for
our fragile brothers and
sisters to whom
we minister.

It is sometimes suggested that caring is the central activity of nursing. I do not disagree with that concept but prefer to add the adjective *compassionate* to a nurse's caring. Based on this perception I wrote a book entitled *The Nurse's Calling: The Spirituality of Compassionate Caregiving.* I believe that one can care about many things and for many reasons, but such caring may not always contain within it the virtue of compassion. For nurses compassion must be the catalyst for and the spiritual undergirding of our caring for the ill and the infirm. Jesus taught us, *"You must love your neighbor as yourself"* (*Matthew* 19:19); he also taught us, through the ministry of His disciple Paul, to *"clothe"* ourselves *"with compassion"* (*Colossians* 3:12), so that *"whatever"* we do *"in word or deed"* will be done *"in the name of the Lord Jesus"* (*Colossians* 3:17). Thus it follows that in loving our neighbor, in serving our neighbor, in caring for our sick neighbor, we must do so not only with caring but with a posture of compassionate caring.

In commenting on the above passage from Paul's Letter to the Colossians, scripture scholar Ivan Havener notes that such "positive admonitions" were given to the Colossians as new Christians, as God's chosen ones: "God's chosen ones are those," he observed, "who are in Christ, holy and beloved, even as he is, and this requires putting on clothes of virtue."[1] Havener adds that Paul "cites a catalog of virtues which should be the dress of the Christian life."[2]

But in what does this virtue of compassion exist? What does it mean for nurses? And how can compassion be lived out in the day-to-day practice of our profession?

Michael Downey defines compassion as follows:

[T]he capacity to be attracted and moved by the fragility, weakness and suffering of another. It is the ability to be vulnerable enough to undergo risk and loss for the good of another. Compassion involves a movement to be of assistance to the other, but it ineluctably entails a movement of participation in the experience of the other in order to be present and available in solidarity and communion. Compassion requires sensitivity to what is weak and/or wounded, as well as the vulnerability to be affected by the other. It also demands action to alleviate pain and suffering. One's deepest inner feelings should always lead to outward compassionate acts of mercy and kindness.[3]

Michael Downey's understanding of compassion is one that can truly be embraced by nurses. Initially, Downey suggests that compassion consists of a person having the "capacity to be attracted and moved by the fragility, weakness and suffering of another."[4] Do we not often hear nurses admit that they chose nursing precisely because of such an "attraction." Debbie, a young graduate working in pediatric oncology, commented, "I know that I'm called to care for people. When I was little I always took care of my sick dolls. Now, I'm doing it with real dolls! It's special, nursing! When someone is hurting or weak or sick from some disabling thing, they need us. And that means a lot to me, to be needed as a nurse."

The second sentence in Michael Downey's definition specifies a compassionate person having the ability to "be vulnerable enough to undergo risk and loss for the good of another."[5] This also is a critical characteristic of nurses. In most caregiving situations nurses are faced with experiences in which they become close to their patients; nurses may spend hours providing support and hope and courage for fragile individuals, knowing full well that the relationship could well be temporary, especially as a patient's disease escalates to a terminal or end-of-life stage.

Some years ago I did hospital chaplaincy training at a major research-oriented medical center. My assigned unit was pediatric oncology and HIV infection. Whereas a few terminally ill children died on the unit, most returned to their homes and families for their final hours. Although this was, of course, supported by the hospital staff, the pediatric nurses told me that it was hard for them because they often did not have a chance to say goodbye to little ones whom they had grown to love over the course of treatment. The nurses asked if the hospital chaplaincy department would plan a general memorial service for the pediatric unit; this would give the staff a chance to mourn the loss of the children who had died during the past year. The pediatric nurses were aware of their personal vulnerability and the deep need to grieve the loss of their precious small patients.

Next, Michael Downey asserts, the compassionate individual must not only seek to "be of assistance to the other" but must actually participate in the "experience of the other" and "be present and available in solidarity and communion."[6] Erin, one of my students, told a wonderful story of assisting with a painful debridement of a wound. The patient, who was trached, kept mouthing the words for pain medication and had tears in her eyes, yet no one seemed to notice. Thus Erin, feeling deeply her patient's pain, stepped forward and asked the physician to stop the procedure until pain medication could be administered. Erin reported that after the procedure was completed the patient wrote her a note saying, "thank you, for being there for me today."

Downey's definition of compassion also includes requisites that one be sensitive to "what is weak and/or wounded" (as well as being vulnerable) and that one take action "to alleviate pain and suffering."[7] This characteristic is the heart of nursing; it is the mission of all nurses to care for the weak and the wounded, to alleviate pain and suffering. Because these virtues characterize the vocation of all nurses, it is difficult to choose one example. As discussed in the section, "The Mysticism of Everyday Nursing," in Chapter 8, often a nurse's caring is a hidden ministry known only to the nurse and his or her patient. One nursing group, however, whose caregiving encompasses many acts of hidden ministry yet whose ministry also overtly reaches out to some of the weakest and most vulnerable members of the human family immediately comes to mind. That is the Frontier Nursing Service (FNS), founded by Mary Breckenridge in 1925, to go forth on horseback to care for poor mothers and babies in the backwoods and hollows of rural Kentucky.[8] Although, FNS nurses have now switched from horses to jeeps or other four-wheel drive vehicles to visit needy mothers and children, they continue to minister especially to the poor and the weak; these nurses truly witness the vulnerability to be "affected" by the needs of the other.

Finally, Michael Downey observed, in his understanding of compassion, that it is a person's "deepest inner feelings" that must "lead to outward compassionate acts of mercy and kindness."[9] In essence, this last statement in Downey's definition of compassion is an extension of the opening characteristic that dealt with one's being able or having the "capacity" to be moved by fragility and weakness of another. It is precisely in the sense that Michael Downey understands compassion as encompassing an individual's "deepest inner feelings" being the catalyst for "acts of mercy and kindness" that we consider nursing not only a profession but also a vocation. From the time of Florence Nightingale, who wrote of nursing, "A new art and science has been created ... and with it a new profession, so they say; we say calling,"[10] to the contemporary practicing nurse, our profession is considered by most as a spiritual calling to serve ill brothers and sisters.

Donna, a 27-year-old nurse practicing in the oncology department of an urban medical center, asserted, "Nursing is definitely a compassionate vocation, a calling that you feel in your heart to serve. For me it's a calling from God. It's why you rotate shifts, even when you're tired. You skip meals when a patient needs you. You stay over after shift report if the staff is really tight and the patients need care. You don't punch a clock and say 'Okay, time for me to leave. Bye! There's somebody bleeding over there, but it's time for me to go.' Nursing isn't like that. Nursing is definitely a vocation."

In his book, *The Conspiracy of Compassion: Breathing Together for a Wounded World,* Paulist Father Joseph Nassal observed that, "when we breathe deeply, allowing God to restore life from within us, our capacity for compassion increases," and "When we grow in our capacity for compassion, we will be less prone to judge and more prepared to serve; more reluctant to condemn and more ready to console; more intent on decreasing the room in our hearts for fear even as we make room for the infinitely spacious compassion of our God in Jesus Christ."[11] "Ironically," Father Nassal adds, "when we increase our capacity for compassion, we make room for joy. For when the gift of compassion is given to another, we discover that we receive so much more."[12]

This also is a wonderful message and validation for nurses. Our lives and our practice must be about compassion; compassion is central to everything we do in nursing practice. How blessed we are as nurses to know that as we continue our day-to-day nursing and as our compassion grows, so also our joy will grow. Most importantly, there will be more room in our hearts for the indwelling of the compassionate Lord of our hearts.

A WOUNDED WORLD

God is our refuge and strength, a very present help in trouble.
Therefore we will not fear though the earth should change, though
the mountains shake.

                                                            Psalm 46:1–2

Jesuit Richard J. Clifford comments that Psalm 46 was written for the people of Israel who were "terrified by the prospect of a collapsing world.... Because God is present at the ordered world's center," he adds, "the psalmist is confident that there will be no unleashing of ... unruly forces."[13] There are some people today who worry about or even predict the "collapsing" of our world, a world wounded by war, by poverty, by sickness, by injustice, and by a variety of other ills that affect the well-being of humankind. In the opening paragraphs of this chapter, the concept of compassion as a central virtue of nursing was discussed. Can such nursing compassion be viewed as an antidote to a "wounded world"? Can we nurses, by living out our call to care for the fragile and the weak, the ill and the injured, serve as loving witnesses to heal a wounded world?

Writing, in 1911, of the great patroness of nursing "Catherine of Siena," English poet Algernon Swinburne seemed to think so. In his famous poem, Catherine of Siena, Swinburne observed, "Then in her sacred saving hands, she took the sorrows of the lands...and in her virgin garment furled, the faint limb of a wounded world."[14] Catherine of Siena lived from 1347 to 1380, only a span of 33 years, but her era was a time of great suffering and upheaval in Europe. The continent was ravaged by the presence of poverty and infectious diseases such as leprosy; most notable, however, was the occurrence of the "Black Plague" epidemic that swept across the land, leaving thousands dead or maimed in its wake. Catherine is described as having been devoted to the poor and the sick, especially lepers, and when Siena was overcome with the plague, she is said to have "walked night and day in the (hospital) wards, only resting a few hours now and then in an adjacent house."[15] In describing Catherine's compassion for the sick, Blessed Raymond of Capua wrote, "Catherine was wonderfully compassionate to the wants of the poor, but her heart was even more sensitive to the sufferings of the sick."[16] Catherine's commitment and compassion for the sick were so well recognized in her own city that after her death, "the citizens of Siena took the very practical point of view of erecting a monument in her memory by rebuilding the hospital in which her work had been done ... (it) stands as a memorial to her unselfish devotion to her fellow men and women...particularly for those who were in saddest need of care."[17]

Some of contemporary society's closest imitators of Catherine of Siena might be identified as those nurses who, especially during the initial onset of the pandemic, undertook the care of persons living with HIV infection and AIDS. AIDS has become the plague of the 20th and 21st centuries in our wounded world. In the early days its aura of contagion, as the Black Plague of Europe, was very frightening to those who ministered to persons suffering from the disease. Nevertheless, an army of compassionate nurses risked caring for this fragile and often stigmatized group of brothers and sisters. One AIDS nurse observed the following:

> I'm not afraid; I can't be; these patients need my care and my caring. Maybe it's a risk. I don't know but I know that I'm called to care for them as a nurse. That's what nursing is all about; it's about risking and caring and being present to sick

people, regardless of what their illness is. I feel blessed to be a nurse during this epidemic when the need for caring is so great. I thank God for the gift of my nursing abilities and for the grace to share them with those who need me.

THE POWER TO HEAL

Then Jesus called the twelve together and gave them power and authority…to cure diseases, and he sent them out to proclaim the kingdom of God and to heal.

Luke 9:1–2

Discussing the "apostolic mission" of Jesus' followers, scripture scholar Jerome Kodell observes that Jesus is now preparing his disciples for their future ministry: "He shares with them his own power and authority" and adds the instruction that "they are to imitate the Master in taking nothing along. Christ's disciples must concentrate on the mission, not their own needs."[18] This is noted in the statement recorded in the Gospel of *Luke* (9:3), which follows that cited above: "Take nothing for your journey, no staff, nor bag, nor bread, nor money, not even an extra tunic." "Jesus," however, "equips the apostles with his own spiritual authority to expel demons, to cure the sick and to proclaim the kingdom of God…. Trusting in God, the apostles must rely on local hospitality for necessities."[19]

These scripture passages might have been written directly for nurses who have been called by the Lord to cure and to heal and in so doing also proclaim the Kingdom of God by their caring ministries. As in Kodell's commentary, nurses are also called to "take nothing with them" but to "concentrate on their mission and not their own needs." This biblical teaching is relevant for contemporary nursing practice. Nurses of the 21st century may at times be beset by many of their own concerns related to such issues as family, housing, or financial constraints, yet these concerns must be left behind when arriving at a patient care setting. Nurses cannot bring personal concerns into the nurse–patient interaction for they must, as Jesus taught, concentrate on their mission, the mission of nursing the sick, rather than on their own needs or worries. Nurses must, when engaged in nursing, whether in clinical practice, administration, management, research, or teaching, trust in the Lord who has equipped us with His "spiritual authority" to heal.

An intensive care unit (ICU) nurse, Pam, spoke about the difficulty and yet also the necessity of leaving "personal baggage" at home when coming to work in the intensive care unit:

It's hard some days. You have a sick child, or your husband has some issues at his job, or the plumber needs to come fix some pipes before the winter and it's going to cost an arm and a leg, but you have to let that stuff go when you come in [to work]. You have these really sick patients who are fragile and afraid, and you have families who are 'spacing out' over what's happening to their family member, and you have to give them 100%. Your head can't be someplace else when you're working in the unit; all of you, body, mind, and soul, has to be there in this nursing. I guess it's like that in all nursing but I can see it so clearly since I've been working in ICU. Every day you have a mission; sometimes it seems like a mission impossible, but with God's help you can make it through the shift and leave feeling that you really have accomplished a mission of healing.

Pam added, "That's the real gift of being a nurse; knowing that you can get past your own needs and help heal others who have more needs than you."

What a magnificent gift nurses have been given by the Lord's commission to His followers to care for the sick: the "power...to heal." In the past, and perhaps even sometimes today, the concept of "healing" is associated with the role of the physician. We've often heard the cliché, "doctors heal; nurses care." In an earlier era there may have been some truth to that maxim when it came to the physical diagnosis and prescription of treatment. Currently, however, I'm sure my nurse practitioner colleagues would strongly disagree with such a generalization as they also diagnose and prescribe in their practices.

Even for nurses who are not practitioners, however, and even in the early days of the profession of nursing, nurses were blessed with the ability to "heal" broken hearts and broken spirits with their compassion and caring. That is what Pam's story of ICU nursing is reminding us: nurses' magnificent ability to heal by being fully present to the needs of their patients, especially those who are, as Pam noted, "fragile and afraid."

One research assignment, when I was serving in the U.S. Navy Nurse Corps Reserve, was to explore the needs and anxieties of ventilator-dependent patients and their families in the ICU of a Naval Hospital. Because I had never actually been an ICU nurse, I asked to spend a week as a "corpsman," working with and observing the staff, to have a better understanding of what exactly ICU nurses did and what needs of the patients seemed most significant.

When I completed my week of observing and learning, I wrote a letter to the ICU staff to express my gratitude and awe at the loving care I had seen exemplified in the nursing of their patients, including those who were comatose and seemingly unresponsive. I told the staff that my greatest inspiration was the fact that they never seemed to lose sight of the "patient" amid the myriad tubes and wires and lines sustaining life in this highly technological ICU environment. It was both amazing and humbling to watch young corpsmen and nurses carrying on a running conversation with a comatose patient: "Good morning, Mr. Jones. It's a beautiful morning today. It's about 8 o'clock and I'm going to be your nurse today. My name is Ensign Gallegher. I'm going to take your vital signs first, then I'll suction out your trach so that you'll feel better and then get you washed up." And, on and on, the conversations would go throughout the staff member's interaction with his or her patient. I asked the nurses about this, and they explained that because we never know how much a comatose patient may hear or understand or what stimulation may help, all the ICU staff were taught to talk to their patients as if they could understand every word. It was quite touching to watch. It also reminded me that these staff members were truly "standing on holy ground" as they sought to heal their critically ill patients.

REMOVE YOUR SANDALS

Remove the sandals from your feet, for the place on which you are standing is holy ground.

Exodus 3:5

Moses was keeping the flocks...and he came to Horeb, the mountain of God. There an angel of the Lord appeared to him in a flame of fire out of a bush...Moses said: "I must turn aside and...see why the bush is not burned up." When the Lord saw that he had turned aside to see, God called to him out of the bush, "Moses, Moses!...Come no closer! Remove the sandals from your feet, for the place on which you are standing is holy ground." (Exodus 3:1-5).

One commentary on the "Burning Bush" scripture notes that in the passage, "God calls and equips his man...Moses is actually at Sinai (Horeb), the very place where he will later receive the law, when God's call comes. God has a stupendous commission for Moses...to lead his people to freedom."[20]

In an earlier book I cited the Exodus story of Moses and the burning bush as well, modeling "the spiritual posture of nursing." God instructed

Moses that when he stood before Him, the very earth on which he was standing was holy. "When the nurse clinician, nurse educator, nurse administrator or nurse researcher stands before a patient, a student, a staff member or a study participant, the ground on which the nurse is standing is holy. For it is here, in the act of serving a brother or sister in need, that the nurse truly encounters God. God is present in the nurse's practice of caring just as surely as He was present in the blessed meeting with Moses so many centuries ago."[21] Thus it is imperative for nurses to figuratively "remove the sandals from their feet," to walk humbly and gently, as a barefoot person might, into the presence of those to whom they would minister.

Perhaps one of the best examples I have personally experienced of needing to "remove the sandals" from my own feet was when I began an internship in hospital chaplaincy several years ago. Although I came to the program with many years of both clinical nursing and nursing research experience, my chaplain supervisor said, "Now you have to begin at the beginning to learn to be a chaplain; you need to leave your nurse's cap in the trunk of the car" (figuratively, of course, as I've not actually worn a nurse's cap in years!). It was difficult, at first, but I understood that mandate from my supervisor. In a way it was like "removing the nursing shoes" from my feet and going barefoot into the experience of hospital chaplaincy. I had to recognize that I was now, just as when I first began my nursing education, standing on new "holy ground" before the Lord and I needed to come to that place open and unencumbered by preconceived notions and concerns, to come, as ICU nurse Pam described, without "personal baggage."

The same suggestion can apply for every new nursing situation we enter; no two patients, no two care situations are exactly the same, yet each presents us the blessed opportunity of "standing on holy ground." Hopefully, we will not fail to "feel" the holiness of the ground on which we are standing because of the encumbrance of some unnecessary "shoes"!

A GENTLE AND QUIET SPIRIT

Let your adornment be the inner self with the lasting beauty of a
gentle and quiet spirit, which is very precious in the Lord's sight.

1 Peter 3–4

A scriptural commentary on the above passage from the First Letter of Peter notes that the teaching was probably directed to women of the era who were being advised to shun "the extravagant ornamentation, clothing, and hair-styling which seemed to be the passion of the day.

Their beauty is in the purity of their chaste behavior, an interior beauty of the heart and a gentle disposition."[22] In current society's emphasis on self-image, self-indulgence, and self-centeredness, I prefer to emphasize the beauty and in fact uniqueness of a "gentle and quiet spirit." Perhaps that was the norm for many women some years ago; now I fear that it can be more often the exception rather than the rule. However, over and over in the tender and poignant stories of nurse–patient interactions that my students relate I find echoes of Peter's emphasis on a "gentle and quiet spirit."

One such experience was described by Judy, who explained why it was important not to judge patients from listening to someone else's perspective: "One day at morning report, everyone just rolled their eyes when they heard what patient I was assigned to that day. Mr. Walker was an older gentleman that all the staff avoided because they said all he ever did was complain and grouch about everything; nobody wanted to go in his room because you couldn't get out without a list of complaints. They told me 'Good luck with this one!'"

Judy continued, "I have to confess that I was not anxious to go see what Mr. Walker had to complain about that morning. But, then I decided that I wasn't going to judge him from morning report. I was going to take a positive approach. I thought maybe a gentle laid-back way of interacting with the man might make him not angry and defensive. So, I went into his room smiling and quietly told him that I was happy to be his nurse today but before we began any morning care I wondered if there was anything he needed or that I could get him. Did he have a good breakfast? Was he in any pain? Did he have a good night?"

Judy admitted, "My patient looked kind of surprised and also kind of wary, with all my questions about whether he needed anything; he probably knew what kind of a reputation he had with the nursing staff. But," Judy continued, "after taking care of a few small problems we got on with morning care and everything went smoothly. I kept trying to let Mr. Walker say how things should go so that he wouldn't feel so out of control."

Judy concluded, "As I was leaving Mr. Walker reached out for my hand and said 'I want to thank you for taking care of me today; you really treated me like a human being. You're a good nurse!'" Judy added, "I think that was the best thing a patient had ever said to me; I'm so glad I tried a gentle approach and didn't make a judgment just because of what other people said."

Supportive of Judy's patient care experience is the perception of the late John Cardinal O'Connor who was, some years back, actively involved in ministering to AIDS patients. From that experience the Cardinal reported that he found the most important approach in caring for the sick was "spiritual gentleness."[23]

I became fascinated by the concept of spiritual gentleness and explored it in some depth in the literature. I also questioned a group of 15 practicing nurses to obtain their understanding of the meaning of the concept in day-to-day nursing activities. Most of the nurses had no difficulty sharing their understanding of spiritual gentleness; responses included (among others) the following statements:

> "Spiritual gentleness is a quality shown by the nurse who believes she has been called to care for others in the way Jesus taught, kindly, non-judgmentally and with a soft touch."

> "Spiritual gentleness passes from the spiritual center of one human being to another."

> "Spiritual gentleness is intertwined with the concept of caring as the core of the nursing model."

> "Spiritual gentleness evokes feelings of understanding and acceptance; it is rooted in the frailty of our humanness."

> "I personally see spiritual gentleness in nursing as a way to connect with my own feelings and beliefs about spirituality and my commitment to the nursing profession."[24]

All the nurses questioned were able to recall patient interactions in which an approach of spiritual gentleness was the catalyst for positive responses on the part of the person being cared for. "In this era of hi-tech, fast-paced health care and health promotion, nurses desperately need to reaffirm their heritage of spiritual gentleness: a heritage rich with the charism of prayerful devotion to caring for the sick; a heritage characterized by tenderness and empathy in ministering to the ill and the infirm."[25]

A MINISTRY OF COMPASSION: THAT ALL MAY HAVE LIFE

I come that they may have life, and have it abundantly.

John 10:10

In chapter 10 of the Gospel of John, the evangelist describes Jesus as "The Good Shepherd" who "calls his own sheep by name and leads them"(10:3). John, in quoting the Lord, reports that Jesus, as the "Good

Shepherd," assured his followers, "I am the gate. Whoever enters by me will be saved, and will go in and come out and find pasture. The thief comes only to steal and kill and destroy. I come that they may have life and have it abundantly" (John 9–10).

In this metaphorical passage, Jesus is telling His followers that "he intends to defend them against thieves and robbers"... that he wishes all those "listening to his voice" to "come into one fold. Jesus will effect all this because he is the 'Good Shepherd', loved by the Father because he will lay down his life for his sheep."[26] Jesus is willing to surrender His life that His followers might have life and *have it abundantly.*

This chapter began with discussing the centrality of the concept of compassion in the practice of nursing; it is fitting that it end by describing all of nursing as a ministry of compassion following the metaphorical teaching of Jesus as the "Good Shepherd," willing and ready to lay down His life for His sheep. Although, except in situations such as that of military nursing, nurses generally do not have to think about physically being willing to lay down their lives for their patients, they often need to do so figuratively. What I'm thinking of is the many stories nurses have told me about laying down the needs of their lives: for example being so tired they didn't think they could "walk another step" until a bleeding patient was admitted for emergency surgery or so hungry they could "eat a horse," until a fresh post-op patient's blood pressure suddenly crashed or so stressed they just wanted a few quiet minutes to "take a deep breath" until a frantic family member said, 'Please won't you talk to me?' In each of these cases, the nurses lovingly and willingly lay down their fatigue, their hunger, their stress to be present to the patient or family seeking their help.

For our military nurses the possibility of laying down one's life can sometimes be more literal than figurative. Although I have never served in an active duty military nursing capacity, I have had the honor of wearing, for 8 years, the Blue and Gold of the U.S. Navy Nurse Corps Reserve. During that time I met a number of nurses who had served on the USNS hospital ships, *Sanctuary* and *Comfort,* during the Vietnam era. Although these nurses were often loathe to talk about specific combat experiences, small glimpses into their military nursing lives gave me an incredible feeling of awe and respect for the risks they had taken, in an almost matter-of-fact manner; the risks were, it seemed, simply part of their duty to God, to country, and to their commitment to military nursing.

Sometimes there was even a little fun in the military nursing stories I heard. One highly ranked Air Force nurse, who sported a veritable "fruit salad" of brightly colored ribbons on her dress uniform, told of her helicopter being shot down over Vietnam on the way to care for some wounded soldiers. She said wryly, "I was actually relieved we got shot down because I was getting so nauseated, I was afraid I was going to be sick in the helo." Her stomach never did learn to fly comfortably in a helicopter!

An army nurse told about how while stationed in Vietnam, her sleeping tent suddenly came under heavy mortar fire in the middle of the night. She and her nurse roommate had no time to get fully outfitted so they ran, in flannel pajamas and "bunny slippers" sent from home, one grabbing a helmet and the other a flak vest. Their hope was that if either was hit with flying mortar it would land on the head of the nurse wearing the helmet or the chest of the nurse wearing a flak vest.

Both of these military nurses laughed when relating their stories but underneath the humor were very much aware that their lives had indeed been at risk in the combat experiences. They had been willing to lay down their lives for their care of the young soldiers, marines, sailors, and airmen involved in the conflict.

This chapter has been about nurses entering sacred spaces and being "clothed with compassion." The nurses' stories reflect the truth, the reality, and the blessedness of that compassion. No commentary can speak more loudly or more clearly than the anecdotes describing compassion in nursing practice as articulated by the nurses themselves. These nurses are a gift to a wounded world, they have "removed their sandals" to have "the power to heal"; they have approached their caring with a "gentle and quiet spirit" to carry out their "ministry of compassion."

A NURSE'S PRAYER FOR A COMPASSIONATE HEART

(Jesus) had compassion for them and cured the sick.

Matthew 14:14

Dear Lord Jesus, Your ministry to the sick and suffering was graced by the blessing of a compassionate heart. Teach me to be guided by Your compassion as I care for frightened and fragile brothers and sisters in my nursing, the ill and infirm. Help me to become an instrument of Your tender compassion that my nursing might bring healing of body and spirit to those who sit in sorrow and suffering. Let me be always a caring and compassionate nursing minister. Amen.

5 With Steadfast Devotion: Committed to Caring

When he came and saw the grace of God, he rejoiced, and he exhorted them all to remain faithful to the Lord with steadfast devotion.

Acts 11:23

COMMITTED TO CARING

Lord Jesus,
Whose very life was
a commitment to caring,
guide your nurses in our
precious commitment
to care.

Guide your nurses in our
commitment to care
with courage and
compassion;

Guide your nurses in our
commitment to care
with tenderness and
mercy;

Guide your nurses in our
commitment to care
with kindness and
understanding;

Guide your nurses in our
commitment to care
with gentleness and
love;

Guide your nurses in our
commitment to care
with an open mind
and
an undivided heart.

Dear Lord, let Your nurses
never forget the gift and the blessing
and the grace that is our call to
a commitment of caring.

In the previous chapters words from scripture reminded nurses of their holy calling, supported the concept of nursing as ministry, taught the importance of sharing God's gifts, and exhorted those who serve the sick to lives of compassion and caring. With this profound and powerful grounding for the vocation of nursing, we can now reflect on the day-to-day carrying out of our ministry "with steadfast devotion."

In an earlier book I described the concept of devotion as the "charism" of nursing.[1] I explained devotion as "giving oneself over to someone or something out of permanent conviction,"[2] and cited the gentle Saint Francis De Sales who taught that any vocation was blessed when "united with devotion."[3] Francis explained that true devotion "not only does no injury to one's vocation or occupation, but on the contrary adorns and beautifies it...every vocation becomes more agreeable when united with devotion."[4]

The importance of devotion in nursing is also highlighted in the famous Nightingale quote, cited so frequently to describe her understanding of the profession:

Nursing is an art; and if it is to be made an art, it requires as exclusive a devotion, as hard a preparation as any painter's or sculptor's work. For what is having to do with dead canvas or cold marble compared with having to do with the living body; the temple of God's spirit.[5]

But what exactly does this concept of devotion, especially "exclusive devotion" that is steadfast, mean in the daily lives of nurses? As an academician I have for many years witnessed the proclaiming of devotion to the nurse's calling by young students. Some time ago our school's third-year students renamed their moving "Capping Ceremony" to "Commitment to Nursing Ceremony." The students do still receive the "cap" of the school of nursing. After the ceremony, however, their "nurse's caps" generally grace the tops of their computers rather than their heads. The focus of the ceremony, nonetheless, is on commitment, on devotion to duty in future nursing practice. This commitment theme is reiterated 2 years later when, immediately before graduation, the senior students receive another symbol of their professional covenant at the school's "Pinning Ceremony." At both of these rituals, as well as at graduation itself, one hears beautiful and poignant talks and prayers, a central concept of which is always devotion to nursing, devotion to living out the call to care for the ill and the infirm.

This chapter explores how God's strength and shelter support nurses in their devotion to duty, how His grace, His gifts, and His steadfast love guide and encourage us in our nursing ministry of caring.

WALK HUMBLY

He has told you ... what is good ... to do justice, and to love kindness, and to walk humbly with your God.

Micah 6:8

A first step in living out our nursing call of devotion to caring for the sick is to put ourselves in a place of right relationship with Lord, a place of humility. The 8th century Prophet Micah taught that God really only asks three things of His people: to be just, to be loving, and to be humble. In the contemporary nursing world the concepts of justice and love are surely considered desirable practitioner virtues; that of humility, however, is not always viewed as a characteristic to be treasured. And yet humility is central to our lives as Christians. Humility, William Shannon observes, "is rooted in the truth of reality (and) a deep awareness of our limitations ... in the presence of the all-holy God."[6] "It leads us," Shannon adds, "to a profound sense of total dependence on God and an ardent desire to do God's will in all things."[7]

Nurses are taught to value such attributes as intelligence, skill, leadership ability, professionalism, and caring. A "good" nurse is seen as one who is well versed in medical and nursing knowledge, capable of carrying out complex therapeutic interventions, and responsive to the psychosocial and spiritual needs of patients and families. A great deal of professional acumen is expected of today's practicing nurses. Among the desired attitudinal and behavioral characteristics expected of modern day nurses, nonetheless, humility is not generally considered a primary requisite.

Humility is a tricky virtue; as soon as you believe you've got it, you don't! I imagine we've all heard or perhaps even personally expressed the joking phrase, "I'm proud of my humility," a classic spiritual oxymoron. Humility is, simply put, just plain hard to get a handle on. Spiritual writers such as William Shannon tell us about humility and how it manifests in our relationship to God. But few theologians or pastors can tell us how to achieve it.

As I was thinking about the relationship between humility and nursing, a little verse of old, entitled "To be a Nurse," came to mind. The poem's first line advises, "To be a nurse is to walk with God, along the path which the Master trod."[8] The verse goes on to identify various caring and compassionate nursing activities and concludes by suggesting, as Teresa of Avila, that the "Great Physician" is using the nurse as His instrument in ministering to the sick.

To me, this simple poem presents beautifully an undergirding posture of humility for a practicing nurse. The idea of walking "the path" that Jesus "trod" and being used as His instrument in ministering to the ill and infirm reflects a humility of spirit that denies one's own power and ability and relies on those of the Lord.

Meditating on this one poetic thought, "to be a nurse is to walk with God, along the path which the Master trod," reveals the importance of humility in the life of a nurse. Our Master trod a path of self-sacrifice and self-giving to alleviate the suffering of others. He was our role model of humility par excellence. Jesus never once asserted his own will, his own needs, his own desires; his only wish, his only message was "to do the will" of the One who sent him (*John* 6:39). What great humility it takes to totally surrender one's own plans and goals to those of another.

This kind of humility is not easy for nurses who are professionally trained to be in control, to be "on top of things" in caring for our patients. To surrender to God's will in all things is a great challenge, and yet it is what we are asked to do as Christian nurses. Perhaps this is precisely why the poet of old mused that "to be a nurse" one must walk the path that Jesus trod, to walk a path of humility and acceptance.

Pondering the place of humility in nursing also brings to mind an article, published anonymously some years ago, entitled "The Nurse's Mass." In the work, nursing activities are likened to those of a priest at the altar. The author speaks movingly of the great gift a nurse receives in being able to minister to the Lord in caring for "the least" of His brethren. The nurse's humility before this blessing is reflected in the nurse author's comments, such as "Lord, I am not worthy... I shall never cease to marvel at my gift;[9]" "I have nothing to give for what have I, that He did not first give me?;[10]" "I must keep my own personal troubles and indecision to myself, so that I will not burden others;[11]"and "My God I thank Thee for all Thou hast done for me, and in return for all Thy mercies, here are my hands, for which there will be no task too lowly."[12]

Sister Sarah, a dear friend, exemplifies for me the lived reality of humility in nursing. Sister Sarah has, for many years, been practicing nursing in a developing country. The people she serves, the culture of the land, even the language are not her own; nevertheless, she has embraced the community and owned it in a spirit of love, gentleness, and humility. Sister Sarah has spent her entire nursing career learning about and responding to the unique concerns and needs of the ill and infirm in her adopted country. Even after many years she might still be considered by some a "foreigner," and yet she deeply loves and appreciates her mission country and the patients that have now become her own. This kind of humble ministry is not easy for American nurses, but it is surely the Christian path that Jesus taught when he said, "Go therefore and make disciples of all nations" (*Matthew* 28:19).

THIS EXTRAORDINARY POWER

We hold this treasure in clay jars, so that I may be made clear that
this extraordinary power belongs to God and does not come from us.

2 Corinthians 4:7

The concept of Christians as "clay jars," or in some translations as "earthen vessels," has long been one of my favorite scripture passages. It is sometimes described as the "paradox" of ministry. We are to proclaim with our lives the love and compassion of Jesus, yet we can only do so if the "light of the knowledge of God," communicated through his Divine Son, is in our hearts. The paradox, however, is that this precious light is contained within the fragile earthen vessel of a human person. This is so that the "power" that informs and flows from our ministry is recognized as being "of God and not from us" (*2 Corinthians* 4:7).

As a nurse I find the "earthen vessel" analogy very comforting. I believe that is because we nurses have, in fact, a significant pastoral responsibility as part of our caregiving. This has been true from the days of our founder Florence Nightingale who once wrote, "When each morning comes, I kneel down before the Rising Sun and only say: 'Behold the handmaid of the Lord.' "[13]

Since the era of the late 1970s and early 1980s especially, nurses have begun to more directly acknowledge their patients as composed of body, mind, and spirit and thus requiring physical, psychosocial, and spiritual assessment and care. As a result of this heightened awareness, the concepts of holistic health care and holistic nursing were introduced as central to our practice. Nurses, thus, accepted a mandate to minister to their patients' spirits as well as to their bodies and their minds.

Caring for patients' spirits, conducting spiritual assessments and providing spiritual care, is not a ministry that comes easily to all nurses. For many of us, the provision of spiritual care by nurses was not included as a part of our nursing education. This was considered a ministry better left to those formally trained in pastoral care such as a priest, minister, or rabbi. A nurse's religious education and tradition may also make him or her more or less comfortable in carrying out such activities as spiritual assessment and spiritual care.

The bottom line for all practicing nurses to remember, however, is that these activities of ministering to the spirits of our patients is God's work and not ours. And this knowledge can give us great comfort. Yes, the treasure of our faith is indeed held in "earthen vessels," but that is precisely so that all will know that anything we accomplish is not because of ourselves but only because of an extraordinary power that belongs to God alone.

In *The Nurse's Calling: A Christian Spirituality of Caring for the Sick*, I admitted that I loved the "earthen vessel" scripture because I have always been a "timid soul, ever questioning my own abilities."[14] I explained that while earlier in my life I fretted about that part of my personality, I have now come to "befriend my inadequacies, my *earthen vesselness* for I now realize … that when I am able to accomplish something … it is not of myself but only because of the treasure I hold within."[15]

In some patient situations we face, nurses become acutely aware of being earthen vessels. We may feel totally inadequate in finding the right words to comfort a parent whose child is dying with an inoperable astrocytoma. We are heartbroken and left struggling for hopeful thoughts to share with a young mother whose breast cancer has metastasized to the lungs and liver. And we are shaken to the core of our being on learning that one of our own dear friends has been diagnosed with advanced pancreatic cancer. How, we wonder, will we gain the strength and the courage and the skill to meet the extraordinary needs of such patients? How can we call upon God's extraordinary power within us?

I had an experience of interacting with a mother whose 6-year-old son was dying with stage IV non-Hodgkin's lymphoma. When I first entered the sickroom I felt very insecure about how to open a conversation with this grieving mother who had been spending day and night with her terminally ill child. We began with some general discussion about her son's condition and prognosis; the mother shared the fact that she was aware that her little one's suffering was rapidly coming to an end. At that comment I asked if she would like me to have a member of the hospital's pastoral care staff visit. She replied, "I'd rather talk to you if you have time." It is when faced with requests like this that we, as nurses, need to hang on to our gift of being "earthen vessels" and to trust that the God who has blessed us with the Light of Life within will provide the power and the support and the strength that we need to minister in His Name.

THE LORD IS MY STRENGTH

God, the Lord, is my strength; he makes my feet like the feet of a deer, and makes me tread upon the heights.

Habakkuk 3:19

Biblical scholars do not know a great deal about Habakkuk, the author of a short three-chapter Old Testament book, except that he is believed to be one of the minor prophets of his era. Perhaps the most frequently quoted passage from the prophecy is that contained at the book's end, chapter 3, verse 19: "God, the Lord, is my strength: he makes my feet like the feet of a deer, and makes me tread upon the heights"; other translations of the chapter and verse describe the feet of a deer as "hinds' feet."

The well-known book, referenced in Chapter 3, describing our spiritual journey with the Lord is based on this brief verse of Habakkuk. The work is entitled, *Hinds' Feet on High Places*, and is written by a Christian missionary, Hannah Hurnard.[16] In her moving and powerful allegory, Hurnard takes the Christian along a frequently dangerous and tortuous path in the footsteps of the "Chief Shepherd"; the ultimate goal is that he or she will receive longed for "hinds' feet" to be able to navigate the "high places" of God's heavenly kingdom.[17] Although Hannah Hurnard's allegory describes many fearful experiences that a follower of Jesus must encounter, the real purpose of the work is to demonstrate God's strength and care, to teach and encourage the reader that no matter how difficult the path of life, the Lord will never desert His beloved disciples. One of my favorite passages is that in which the Shepherd assures his follower: "Never for a moment shall I be beyond your reach or call for help, even when you cannot see me."[18]

Pat, a nurse with 25 years of experience in caregiving, explained how God's Word communicated in scripture gave her the strength needed to support a patient and family in great need:

> Annie was a middle-aged woman with a husband and two children who had a great job and a terminal diagnosis of bone cancer. She was in the hospital for long-term care; basically she was there to die. During the time I cared for Annie I spent a lot of time with her family.
>
> The family was despondent because of the potential loss of their loved one. As a result I found that I began distancing myself from Annie and her family because I was unable to deal with the feelings that being with them brought about in myself. I could not truly acknowledge what they were going through. I couldn't even let myself think of Annie as more than a collection of problems some of the time because it was just too overwhelming. And I knew that that wasn't right because Annie and her family needed me.
>
> As I attempted to find resources within myself to better deal, I thought of a particular scripture passage, "Blessed are they who mourn for they will be comforted" (*Matthew* 5:4). Every time I encountered Annie and her family I thought of this passage and it helped me to focus not on my own feelings but on their experiences. I knew that I wouldn't be able to do much for them except just be there. I was able to provide the support that was needed and when Annie died they were at peace with it.
>
> At Annie's funeral her husband came up to me and thanked me for all that I had done. He said, "I felt that I was losing control of everything and you just being there for me and my children, just providing comfort through your presence was so wonderful!"

Pat ended her story with the comment, "I have never forgotten Annie and her family. Whenever I am confronted with a similar difficulty, I think about that scripture and it gives me such strength."

Repeatedly, the nurses' anecdotes shared in this book, as Pat's story, reflect "the Lord" as the nurses "strength." Sometimes the Lord's strength comes to the nurse in prayer, sometimes through reading and meditating on scripture, and sometimes simply from the awareness of God's loving presence in His call to care for "the least of His brothers and sisters." However the Lord's strength is perceived, nurses may trust that in times of trouble, the Lord will "hide" them in the shelter of His loving arms.

IN HIS SHELTER

The Lord is my light and my salvation.... For he will hide me in his shelter in the day of trouble; he will conceal me under the cover of his tent.

Psalm 27:1, 5

In attempting to live out our nursing vocation with, as the theme of this chapter suggests, "steadfast devotion," there will of course be "days of trouble." There will be days when the physical or the emotional or even the spiritual stress of caring for the sick simply gets to us. There will be days when we wonder if all this talk of nursing as a vocation, as a calling from God, is "pie in the sky." Our bodies, our minds, our spirits, or all three together, have just become so fatigued that all we want is to "get through" a shift, to do the basics and go home.

But where really is home? Isn't our true home that place of deep quiet and peace and security that can be found only in the loving arms of our Father in heaven, that place where He will indeed "hide" us in "his shelter in the day of trouble."

In the book *Prayer in Nursing* I quoted Benedictine Mary Clare Vincent who wrote, "A life without prayer doesn't work."[19] I followed Sister Mary Clare's thought with the suggestion that "Nursing without prayer doesn't work."[20] Actually, nurses are among the most prayerful people I know. When I was searching the nursing literature for a history of prayer in nursing, I found that many of our early journals contained beautiful and poignant prayers written by nurses. One example, *"A Prayer for Nurses,"* was published in 1952 and reads in part, "Lord Jesus Christ, source of all health and all healing, be with me this day as I go about among Thy sick committed to my care. Place Thine own wounded hand upon my head that all my strength may come from Thee.... Let me find Thee in all the bruised and hurt whose injuries I mend."[21] Another prayer of the same era, entitled *"A Nurse's Night Prayer,"* contained the moving line, "I looked at my patient, there in his bed, but I felt I was seeing the thorn-crowned head."[22]

As I read these words, written so long ago, I yearn for us to reclaim the powerful prayerful heritage of nursing. Our nurse forebears recognized the importance and even necessity of finding their strength in "His shelter," especially in their "days of trouble." Early nurses, providing care in a much less technologically sophisticated medical world, understood that they must turn to the Lord for support and guidance. This recognition of the value of prayer should be even greater for contemporary nurses practicing in a complex medical–ethical–legal health care system of the third millennium.

Nurses can, as noted earlier, pray in many ways. For some, more formal worship with a community of persons of the same faith tradition, in a house of worship, is especially meaningful. For other nurses quiet personal time with the Lord, either in a church or outdoors in a nature setting, is the desired prayer setting. Prayer can be verbal or mental. One kind of verbal prayer that I always find moving is that put to music. Perhaps it is because I have at different periods in my life sung in choirs and I've always loved the concept and quote attributed to St. Augustine that, "He who sings prays twice." That surely sounds like singing is helping us get the most out of our prayers. I suspect St. Augustine may also have been considering the fact that when we sing prayerful music, we put out emotions as well as our minds deeply into the effort.

A variation on singing prayers, for a patient who is very ill or even for a nurse who is very tired, is listening to sacred music. This can be one of the most comforting and relaxing kinds of prayerful interaction with God that one can engage in. Several parish nurses described the importance of sacred music in the spiritual lives of their patients. Jeanine reported, "Mrs. Conrad says that she likes to listen to gospel music...she feels this helps her connect with God since she can't get out to church as much as in the past." Jeanine added, "I visited Mrs. Conrad...we played music tapes and I prayed with her.... She told me that she loved the music tapes I brought her and listened to them with her family." Kristin noted that one of her patients, Mr. Kearney, told her "he enjoyed listening to [sacred] music because it helped his faith." Michele described the importance of music for a nursing home resident, Mrs. Fitzgerald. Mrs. Fitzgerald "thought [some music I brought her] was very moving. She continued to listen to the music after I left.... She listens to the music over and over. The tapes also facilitated family support and interaction. A group of her family members came one day and listened to the music with Mrs. Fitzgerald." Finally, Michele reported, "Mrs. Fitzgerald told me that the music tapes helped her relate to God, to make a connection with him."

Joan, a geriatric nurse, spoke about the importance of recognizing the blessing of "God's shelter" in the practice of nursing with elders: "Mrs. Shelly has advanced Parkinson's disease; it has crippled her body but she is still in control of her mental faculties. She has spent her life as an active member of her community and has taken pride in her professional accomplishments." But, Joan reported, Mrs. Shelly was currently very depressed and felt very far away from a relationship with God or from His help in coping with her illness and disability.

Joan prayed privately for the Lord's shelter in the midst of caring for Mrs. Shelly. Ultimately, Joan suggested to her patient a comforting psalm of God's care and support; they prayed the psalm together. There appeared to be a very peaceful change in the patient's demeanor following their prayer. Joan commented, "It was only the grace of God working in her. I had not thought about the wording of the psalm when I suggested it; I only knew that I had a feeling the Holy Spirit was guiding me, leading me to that particular psalm."

Joan continued, "[Mrs. Shelly] began to talk about her disease as an obstacle, an obstacle to be overcome to help her in her faith journey. She then began to relate it to other challenges that she had faced at various points in her life. We had a great discussion that day, and as I left she embraced me as well as she could, and said something that I will never forget: 'Thank you for giving me the road map; I knew the way to talk to God, but I needed the map'!"

Joan's map provided to Mrs. Shelly was a wonderful reflection of the provision of God's steadfast love.

GOD'S STEADFAST LOVE

How precious is your steadfast love, O God! All people may take refuge in the shadow of your wings.

Psalm 36:7

It important to accept the fact, however, that it's not always easy for us to see Jesus in all of our patients, especially in those who we might consider "difficult." Yet we have to remember that Our Father loves them just as dearly, just as tenderly as those people in our world whom we honor and respect. An English Benedictine retreat master once told a story to illustrate God's steadfast love that I have never forgotten.

The retreat leader recounted an incident in which a young British schoolmaster was straightening up his classroom at day's end. When he arrived at one particular desk, he noticed that the student, an elementary school boy, had left his copybook behind on the floor. The master sighed deeply as he bent to pick up the book because its dog-eared ink-smudged pages so reminded him of the owner who was, in his opinion, a scruffy inky little boy whom the teacher found very difficult to love.

As the schoolmaster picked up the notebook, a letter from the boy's father slipped out and drifted to the floor, falling open as it went. In refolding the letter the teacher's eyes glanced the salutation: "My dearest, most precious child."

I love that story because it always reminds me that when I am not terribly attracted to one of my patients or even when I myself am feeling a bit on the "inky scruffy" side, spiritually I must remember that I, as well as all of my brothers and sisters in the human family, are to our Father in Heaven His dearest most precious children. What a grace, what a blessing is the unconditional and steadfast love of God!

In this chapter the steadfast devotion of God has been explored as a model for the steadfast devotion He would ask of His nurses. Nurses' devotion is understood as being supported and guided by the loving precept of the Lord to "walk humbly," by God's extraordinary power held in nurses hearts through His presence, by God's strength and shelter always and everywhere available to His nurses, and by God's own steadfast love that in turn directs nurses' steadfast love and care for our patients.

A NURSE'S PRAYER OF COMMITMENT AND CARING

Commit your work to the Lord, and your plans will be established.

Proverbs 16:3

Dear Lord Jesus, whose very life was a commitment to caring, teach me commitment to care for the ill and the infirm. Help me to be graced with the courage of a commitment to care. Help me to practice the tenderness of a commitment to care. Guide me to be kind and understanding in my commitment to care. And let my nursing commitment to care be carried out with an open and loving heart. Above all, Dear Lord, let my work of nursing be always committed to You, the source of my strength and the center of my life. Amen.

6 Made Perfect in Weakness: Blessed Vulnerability

My grace is sufficient for you, for power is made perfect in weakness.

2 Corinthians 12:9

BLESSED VULNERABILITY

Dear Lord of Life,
Your disciple Paul taught that
our power would be made perfect
in weakness.
The world teaches that our power
is made perfect in strength.

Lord Jesus, the moment of Your
greatest weakness, as You hung dying
on a roughhewn cross,
became, also, the moment of Your
greatest power, as You redeemed
humanity from the sins
of the ages.

You chose to be vulnerable, Lord Jesus,
that Your followers might be
powerful.

Grant Your nurses the gift of
blessed vulnerability,
that we might, in turn,
be strong in
our service
to the sick.

As discussed in Chapter 5, for a nurse one of the most significant dimensions of caring is compassion. Compassion has been described as "the quality of relatedness to our world and those in our care."[1] To be a compassionate nurse "requires courage and the willingness to be vulnerable and open to the experience of others."[2] I've occasionally had the response on telling someone I was a nurse, "Oh that's wonderful but I could never do that!" Generally, the person adds something to the effect that they can't stand the sight of blood or don't like being around sick people. Sometimes there are questions such as, "Doesn't listening to sick people's problems all the time get depressing?" or "I can't imagine spending my days in such a gloomy place as a hospital!" or, even worse, "It's good that you can do that but I think I'm just too sensitive to watch people go through all that pain and suffering."

That last thought, especially, always seems like a "back-handed" compliment to me. The person is glad that some of us are "insensitive" enough to be daily witnesses to the pain and suffering of our more fragile brothers and sisters. But isn't this precisely the heart of compassion in nursing as defined above, that is "the courage and the willingness to be vulnerable and open" to the trauma and the stress and sometimes the overwhelmingly sorrowful experiences of our patients.

To be open to the suffering of others, to take on some of their pain by listening and by caring is to be vulnerable. For us, as nurses, however, this is a blessed vulnerability; it is a vulnerability that allows us the precious opportunity to cross over and to stand with those who are in suffering and to try to understand. Our vulnerability allows hurting patients to share some of their burden with someone who cares so they will not feel so isolated and alone in their illness or infirmity.

Very often our personal vulnerability, the vulnerability that allows us to reach out and be open to our patients, is the result of some pain or suffering that has occurred in our own lives. For, as noted in the Gospel of Saint John, it is only after the "grain of wheat" has fallen to the ground and died that that small "grain" may bear fruit.

UNLESS THE GRAIN OF WHEAT FALLS

Very truly, I tell you, unless a grain of wheat falls into the earth and dies, it remains just a single grain; but if it dies it bears much fruit.

John 12:24

The theological interpretation of the above scripture teaches that, "As a planted seed must decay before it sprouts new life, so Jesus must endure death to bring us eternal life."[3] It is suggested further that, "this principle also holds true for [Jesus] disciples, who must die to themselves to receive the fullness of life from God and be channels of life to others."[4] As Jesus will one day be glorified, so His followers are promised eternal life, but the death must occur before resurrection and rebirth.

How compelling this "grain of wheat" scripture passage, penned by the evangelist John, may seem to us as nurses when all is going well, when our work is productive and satisfying, when our families and friends are happy and fulfilled, and when the personal goals we have identified are being accomplished or seem, at least, well on the way to that happening. We are able to say, "life is good," and we have a lightness of heart to match our words. In such a spiritual frame of mind John's teaching, although admired and honored, is relegated to the far distant future. Thus although we have the leisure to consider and perhaps to embrace the message that one day we may suffer, suffer even to death, in order to "bear much fruit," we hasten to add "Not now Lord" to our prayerful meditation on John's words. For, we still have a lot of living to do. If, however, suffering comes to us in the future we'll be ready to accept it. Promise!

But, how do we truly feel when we are faced with a here and now "grain" of "wheat" from our well-ordered lives falling into the ground and dying? Are we, in the midst of an experience of suffering, really able to think about the "fruit" that might be born out of the present pain; are we able to understand and to accept Paul's words, which tell us that God's *grace* is enough and His power will be perfected through our weakness?

I have no doubt that many spiritually mature nurses can indeed understand the grace of weakness, can accept, with a sense of peace and joy, the beauty of a death that will "bear much fruit." Personally, however, I have to confess, and this admission bespeaks volumes in terms of my own lack of holiness, that I generally complain bitterly to the Lord when I am faced with a "death" in my spiritual journey. When a "grain" of my tightly grasped life plan "falls into the earth and dies," I rant and rave at God who does not seem to understand at all what it is I need so badly to survive, to follow Him. How could God be so unfair, so unfeeling? Doesn't He know what He's putting me through? "What kind of God are you," I cry, "to treat me like this"? Then, being Irish, an ethnic group that has elevated guilt to an "art form," I feel terrible for yelling at God. I don't, however, immediately take it all back even if I do say "I'm sorry." I justify my distress by remembering that the great Saint Teresa of Avila is reputed to have once exclaimed to God, "If this is how You treat Your friends, no wonder you have so few of them!"

I recently had a very painful experience of a personal "grain" of my life's "wheat" falling into the ground. As described above, I did not handle it well until I took a fresh look at suffering in terms of the meaning of God's love for us. I was greatly helped by reading a passage from C. S. Lewis' classic work, *The Problem of Pain:*[3]

> When Christianity says that God loves (us), it means that God *loves* (us): not that He has some "disinterested," because really indifferent, concern for our welfare, but that, in awful and surprising truth, we are the objects of His love. You asked for a loving God; you have one. The great spirit you so lightly invoked, the "lord of terrible aspect," is present: not a senile benevolence that drowsily wishes you to be happy in your own way, not the cold philanthropy of a conscientious magistrate, nor the care of a host who feels responsible for the comfort of his guests, but the consuming fire Himself, the Love that made the worlds, persistent as the artist's love for his work and despotic as a man's love for a dog, provident and venerable as a father's love for a child, jealous, inexorable, exacting as love between the sexes.[5]

In describing his understanding of God's love in the midst of human pain and suffering, Lewis adds, "What we would here and now call our 'happiness' is not the end God chiefly has in view: but when we are such that He can love without impediment, we shall in fact be happy."[6]

A BRUISED REED

He will not break a bruised reed or quench a smoldering wick.

Matthew 12:20

In citing the above scripture, Matthew is quoting the Old Testament words of Isaiah who prophesied that God's "chosen servant" would not "break a bruised reed or quench a smoldering wick." It is noted that the prophecy is fulfilled when Jesus "withdraws from his enemies and ministers to the lowly."[7] In the myriad gospel stories of Jesus' healing ministry, we learn how the Lord ministered to the lowly, to those who were poor and suffering; how He healed rather than broke those who were bruised with illness or infirmity (e.g., Peter's mother-in-law ill with a high fever, *Luke* 4:38–39; the paralytic lowered through the roof, *Luke* 5:17–26; the woman with a 12-year hemorrhage, *Luke* 8:43–48; the leper who sought cleansing, *Luke* 5:12–16; the bent-over woman, *Luke* 13:10–17; and the man blind from birth, *John* 9:1–7).

Jesus also brought healing to those in whom the wick of life seemed to be smoldering (Jairus' dying daughter, *Luke* 8:40–42, 51–55; the Roman Official's son who lay critically ill and near death, *John* 4:46–54; the widow's dying son, *Luke* 7:11–17; and a man ill for 38 years, *John* 5:1–9).

The scripture describing the Lord as one who would never break a "bruised reed" or "quench a smoldering wick" is one of my favorite descriptions of Jesus both personally and for my ill and disabled patients. I like to think of God's Divine Son, sent to teach and save us, as embodying not only a great love but also a great gentleness. This scripture especially reminds me of Dante's description of the evangelist/physician Luke as "the scribe of Christ's gentleness" because Luke's gospel focused so much on recording the Lord's mercy to those who were suffering.[8]

For our patients, for example, for an ill elderly person coping with the multiple disabling conditions that may accompany the aging process, the analogy of the "bruised reed and smoldering wick" is most appropriate. As one ages the body can indeed become scarred with a variety of "bruises," and "while one's spirit may still be burning with the desire to serve…," the flame of activity present in earlier years has now become more like the "smoldering wick" than the flaming fire of youth. Thus the knowledge that Jesus, the Servant of the Lord, will treat a "bruised reed" and "smoldering wick" with gentleness and compassion can provide comfort, especially to the older adult facing serious illness and death.[9]

So often we nurses find our patients to be as "bruised reeds" and need to remember the gentleness of our Master and teacher Jesus who would never "break a bruised reed." Sandy, a med-surg nurse, related a touching account of her interaction with Charlie, one of her more fragile patients. She reported, "I had an interaction with one of my patients one day which did not specifically have to do with prayer or spirituality really, but a lot to do with humanity and compassion; it was an indirect display of my faith in my practice. The use of touch can mean so much to fragile patients."

Sandy continued, "This assigned patient was a man in his late sixties. The NAs [nursing assistants] had done his morning care and moved on to their next patients. My patient called for a bedpan and nobody responded to his need. When I got there it was too late. I went and got a basin, clean gown, clean sheets, and promptly cleaned up the patient and his bed again. [While doing this] I just talked to him about the World Series that was going on, as though nothing had happened, to uphold his dignity as much as possible."

Sandy went on, "After I finished I left to get his meds, and when I brought them back, he looked at me and said, 'Thank you, Thank you for being a good nurse and caring; thank you for not treating me like a child while you fixed me up!' I smiled and assured Charlie that it had been no trouble."

Sandy concluded, "My goal as a nurse has always been to see Christ in my patients and treat my patients as I would him; this very thing, this call to serve, is an integral part of living Christian life and, as far as I'm concerned, the life of a nurse."

Sandy had been very gentle with this "bruised reed" who had been committed to her care.

CONTENT WITH WEAKNESS

Therefore I am content with weakness, insults, hardships, persecutions and calamities for the sake of Christ; for whenever I am weak, then I am strong.

2 Corinthians 12:10

The admission of being "content with weakness" that Saint Paul included in his second letter to the new Christians of Corinth was a powerful and humbling confession on the part of the man, once named Saul, who had been a leader in the Jewish community. But Paul's statement was meant to both witness and to teach the young Christian community whose care he cherished. It is suggested that Paul's comment "reveals the truth that divine power is made more evident in human frailty. When Paul is most empty of all human cause for boasting, he is able to identify and testify to the source of his power and strength."[10] "This amazing reversal of all earthly wisdom," it is added, "transforms weakness, distress and mistreatment into powerful evidence of God's presence."[11]

It's not easy for anyone to be "content with weakness," especially in the contemporary American culture when everything with which we are bombarded by the media seems to support the concept of strength and power and being in control of our lives both personal and professional. The social environment of today's society makes it more and more difficult to support and encourage our patients who are facing temporary or sometimes extended periods of physical and/or emotional weakness due to an illness or disability. As with a "bruised reed," however, approaching a weak patient with caring and compassion can go far in helping them to accept and even feel positive about his or her experience of infirmity.

Lisa, a geriatric nurse, described caring for Bill, an 82-year-old gentleman who was frustrated and railing against his current disability related to a diagnosis of multiple sclerosis. Lisa reported, "I had my work cut out for me in caring for him and that was clear from the outset at the gates. He did not seem to think I was old enough or worthy to provide spiritual care for him. Because he was feeling his own weakness so deeply, we spoke about Saint Paul's admission of being 'content with weakness'. Paul struggled and had fear during his years of ministry...and had some awful times while ministering to the Corinthians."

Then Lisa added, "[Bill] said how could he manage when Paul could not even keep it together over the long haul? I acknowledged his comments and acknowledged that Paul did struggle. I pointed out, however, that the Bible provides us many instances where great leaders struggled, but most always came out of their struggle, renewed and stronger in their faith."

Lisa continued, "[Bill] wanted an example; he needed something to improve his outlook so I quoted the only solid passage I could think of: 'What will separate us from the love of Christ? Will anguish, or distress, or persecution, or famine, or nakedness, or peril or the sword? No in all these things we conquer overwhelmingly through him who loved us. For I am convinced that neither death, nor life, nor angels, nor principalities, nor present things, nor future things, nor powers, nor height, nor depth, nor any other creature will be able to separate us from the love of God in Christ Jesus our Lord (*Romans* 8:35, 37–39).'"

After the scripture reading, Lisa noted, "[Bill] was less defensive than I have ever seen him and he clutched his Bible, seeming to be much calmer. He...stated that this would be a good passage for him to reflect on, to help him work out his current feelings of self pity."

In conclusion, Lisa reported, "[Bill] took my hand and we prayed together. I departed feeling that God had graced me enough to be able to reach this man and hopefully help him be somewhat content with his current weakness."

ALL SUFFER TOGETHER

For just as the body is one and has many members...so it is with Christ. For in the one spirit we were all baptized into one body....
If one member suffers, all suffer together.

1 Corinthians 12:12–13, 26

In describing the body of the Church, Paul uses the analogy of the human body, explaining "The body is not identified with any one member, but needs many members cooperating as one. Each believer is a member of the body of Christ."[12] Because, as with the human physiology, all of the parts of a church community are interconnected, pain or disability in one "member" may be felt throughout the entire body. Thus scripture scholar Mary Ann Getty observes, "If one member suffers, every other member suffers, and all other members instinctively supply for the hurt member. Similarly, if one member is given special recognition, all members are more animated because they share in this honor."[13]

The scripture passage from 1 Corinthians 12 that reminds us that if one member of the body suffers, all suffer together brings to mind again the importance of empathy and compassion in nursing. Suffering emotionally with our patients becomes a way of life for nurses actively engaged in the practice of our profession. We always say that we try not to "take our work home," but often, especially if we are working with deeply suffering patients, that's just not possible. I believe Saint Paul was absolutely on target when he noted that if one part of a body, one member of a community, suffers, all share the suffering to some degree.

A poignant and powerful example of Paul's perception of a suffering community was, I believe, the experience of our country, I might dare even say of our world, after the terrorist attacks of 9/11. Virtually everyone in this country can tell you exactly where they were and what they were doing and who they were with on the morning, evening, and night of September 11, 2001. And after an initial attempt to assess the well-being of loved ones who might have been at or near the attack sites in New York, Washington, DC, and Pennsylvania, hearts and minds were immediately filled with sorrow for those others, not personally known, but suffering terribly from the disaster. On that day and the days that immediately followed, America and many countries around the world were united and bonded in suffering as never before. Suddenly differences in age, gender, religion, socioeconomic status, and ethnic background no longer mattered. People needed to communicate with each other, to support each other, to pray for each other, and to share in each other's sufferings. Young people held candlelight vigils, elders offered words of comfort and sympathy, workers flew flags proudly and courageously, parents hugged their children tight, and the world cried and grieved with the victims of the attacks. No one was left untouched or unscarred nor did they want to be. All recognized that in this time of terrible tragedy they not only needed but wanted to suffer together with those who were suffering so much more. Empathy and compassion were the attributes of the days and weeks and months after the attack.

And so with nurses who, pray God, never again see such widespread and violent suffering as that experienced on 9/11, empathy and compassion is the watchword of our days as we suffer with our patients who suffer, cry with our patients who cry, and grieve with our patients who grieve for the lives they once had and may have no longer.

PLANS FOR YOUR WELFARE

For surely I know the plans I have for you, says the Lord, plans for
your welfare and not for harm, to give you a future with hope.

Jeremiah 29:11

Because the Prophet Jeremiah lived in troubled times of war and suffering, a "time of darkness and despair,"[14] he was sensitive, in his writings, to asserting God's ultimate care for his people. Thus he explained carefully in chapter 29 of his prophecy that despite a long period of sorrow and exile, the Lord's ultimate plans for his people were for their "welfare." Jeremiah added God's assurance: "When you call upon me and come to pray to me I will hear you. When you search for me, you will find me; if you seek me with all your heart I will let you find me...and I will restore your fortunes...and I will bring you back to the place from which I sent you into exile" (*Jeremiah* 29:12–14). In this passage the Lord is assuring his people that he "will reverse their fortunes and bring them back to their own land."[15]

Those who are ill or disabled often also believe they are in exile; this is especially true for individuals dealing with chronic or long-term illnesses. Julie, a parish nurse, spoke about one of her patients who felt totally alone and "exiled" in her illness. The patient did not believe that God had any "plans for her welfare." Julie explained, "I met with Ann and it was a battle; she was sick with so many problems, primarily end-stage renal failure."

Julie attempted to support and encourage her patient but was not sure how successful she had been before the patient's death; she finally concluded that the outcome must be left in the hands of God. This happens to us as nurses sometimes. Although this book contains many stories of nurses' magnificently poignant spiritual interactions with patients, we must recognize that we may not always see the fruit of our caring and our ministry.

Julie admitted that immediately after her patient Ann's death she felt dejected, just drained: "not knowing if I did or said the right things, if I made a difference for this person I was trying to help. But then I pulled out my Bible and flipped to the passage that I always lean on, that I always use to renew my strength and hope: 'But I am not alone, because the Father is with me. I have told you this so that you might have peace in me. In the world you will have trouble, but take courage for I have conquered the world.' (*John* 16:33)."

Stories like Julie's, and those of the other nurses included in this chapter, are important because they remind us that as blessed as we nurses are to have been called to this ministry of caring and compassion, we are also weak and we are vulnerable. We become deeply involved with many of our patients and we hurt with them, for them, and we grieve especially if we sometimes believe we have not been able to minister to them as we would wish, that our human caring did not "work" the way we had hoped. It is at these latter times, especially, that we must remember Saint Paul's teaching of the Lord, quoted at the opening of this chapter: "My grace is sufficient for you, for power is made perfect in weakness" (2 *Corinthians* 12:9). This is precisely why Paul also reminded us of the importance of recognizing that we are but "earthen vessels" in order that "it may be made clear that this extraordinary power belongs to God and does not come from us (2 *Corinthians* 4:7)."

A NURSE'S PRAYER FOR STRENGTH IN WEAKNESS

Whoever serves must do so with the strength that God supplies so that God may be glorified in all things through Jesus Christ.

1 Peter 4:11

Dear Lord Jesus, strengthen my service of nursing that I might be an instrument of Your love. You, who so totally embraced fragile humanity, understand the need for the gift of strength in our weakness. I try to embrace the pain and the fear and the sorrow of my frail patients. I don't understand the why of their suffering; help my lack of understanding. Grant me the strength and the faith and the hope to trust in Your will and to lovingly support each patient for whom I care. Amen.

7 ☙ The Winter Is Past: Empowered by Faith

Arise my love, my fair one, and come away; for now the winter is past, the rain is over and gone.

Song of Solomon 2:10–11

ARISE, MY LOVE AND COME

"Arise, my love, my fair one, and come
*   away; for now the winter is past, the*
rain is over and gone. The flowers appear
*   on the earth; the time of singing has come,*
and the voice of the turtle-dove is heard in
*   our land.*
Arise, my love, my fair one, and come
*   Away."*

The Song of Songs 2:10–11; 13

This was the Song she had longed for
*   so deeply;*
this was the summons to come
*   from His throne;*
this was the message she prayed
*   for so fiercely;*
this was the call she desired
*   as her own.*

But the winter of illness
*   was frigid and long;*
savage rains beat down on
*   her soul.*

No flowers or singing appeared
*   in the land;*
no voice which could now
*   make her whole.*

The sunlight was muted with
*   shadow;*
her world blanketed with
*   coldness and chill.*
The poetry of love was an
*   empty verse;*
the music was silent and still.

Vicious winds blew and
*   threatened;*
icy blasts frightened and
*   shocked;*
Yet, He whom her heart
*   loveth;*
had hidden her soul in
*   the cleft of a rock.*

Now the rain is over; the
*   winter is past;*
And the voice of the Beloved
*   calls her at last:*
*   "Arise, my love, my fair one*
*   and come away ... let*
*   me see your face,*
*   let me hear your voice,"*
Let me love you into this day.

For a person who has long been suffering from a chronic or life-threatening illness, the classic and beautiful passage that begins "Arise, my love, my fair one and come away," from the second chapter of the *Song of Songs*, may be both encouraging and comforting, especially in the message, "For, now the winter is past, the rain is over and gone." It may help one for whom the burden of illness and disability seems at times unbearable to understand that if not immediately then one day, the pain, the agony of his or her physical, emotional, and perhaps even spiritual suffering will be ended. At long last there will be a spiritual "light at the end of the tunnel" as it were, and the joy of being in the arms of the Resurrected Christ may be glimpsed.

In a moving mystical interpretation of the *Song of Songs*, Jesuit George Maloney described his understanding of the phrase, "For see, the winter is past, the rains are over and gone," as follows: "Winter is a sign here of the many trials of coldness, darkness and a sense of being close to death."[1] Christ is telling His beloved that suffering is over "through his new life in the Resurrection."[2] Maloney adds, "Nothing outside is life-giving...except the love of Christ. Nothing outside can bring worry, fear, anxiety" for Christ is now with His beloved in a "new and more permanent way."[3]

The *Song of Songs* ends with a second call to the beloved to "come." Maloney interprets this to mean that because Christ has never left His beloved, the call is to "come forth" from a hiding place in the "clefts of the rocks." He wants the beloved "to come to him in a new surrendering way.... Leaving (herself) is like the death of Winter. Coming to the beloved and surrendering more totally to his loving union is to bring spring and summer to full harvest."[4]

Although some question the seemingly overt romanticism of the *Song of Songs*, a Hebrew superlative for "the best song,"[5] it has been accepted into the Christian canon of scripture as "it could easily describe in allegory the love of Christ for the Church, or for the soul of the believer."[6] This allegorical interpretation was advocated early on by such masters of the spiritual life as Bernard of Clairvaux and John of the Cross.[7]

Nurses caring for chronically or seriously ill patients will find in the *Song of Songs* a comforting spiritual assurance that no matter how painful their patients' physical suffering, there is hope and even joy to be found in Christ's promise of a new and eternal life.

I WILL NOT FORGET YOU

Can a woman forget her nursing child, or show no compassion for the child of her womb? Even these may forget, yet I will not forget you. See, I have inscribed you on the palms of my hands.

Isaiah 49:15–16

In commenting on the above words of Isaiah, biblical scholar John Collins asserts that "the most striking" line in the passage is, "Can a mother forget her infant?" "Female experience as well as male," Collins adds, "can serve as analogy for God."[8] Generally, this passage from Isaiah is interpreted as being a metaphor for God's love and tender care for His people whom He remembers with the same attentiveness of a mother toward her child.

Does it ever seem, however, as if God has forgotten some people? Especially those who are sick and suffering? Have you ever looked at a patient, battered and scarred from illness or injury, and wondered, "What does God see in this poor wounded one?" Have you ever looked at yourself, battered and scarred from caring for illness and injury, and wondered, "What does God see in my poor wounded self?"

As I ponder these questions, an old narrative poem, authored by Myra Welch, comes to mind; the work is entitled, *The Touch of the Master's Hand*. In the poem Welch relates a poignant anecdote that describes an auctioneer attempting to initiate some minimal bidding on an old violin. Suddenly, an elderly man comes forth from the crowd, dusts off and tunes the violin, and begins to play a beautiful melody. Now, most of those present recognized the value of the instrument and the bidding increased greatly. A few people, however, admitted that they did not "quite understand" what had "changed" the "worth" of the violin. The auctioneer replied, "The touch of the Master's hand."[9]

And so it is with a fragile patient. The Lord's look on the suffering one and the touch of the "Master's hand" turns a debilitated patient into a beautiful and precious child of God, a child both loved and beloved of the Father. And, it is the "Master's hand" that can also turn our sometimes "dusty" wounded nursing selves into beautiful servants, blessed by our treasured ministry of caring for the sick. We must only be open to the tender loving touch of the "Master's hand."

Eileen, a geriatric nurse, described how she ministered spiritually to Mr. Convey, a 77-year-old gentleman who believed that he had indeed been forgotten by God:

> Although Mr. Convey was baptized a Christian, he does not feel very connected at the present time. He worries about illness among family members but is frank in admitting that he has not the health nor the money to help. He asked if I thought prayer would help? He cried and told me that he wished he felt worthy of the promises that prayer holds, and he believed in the power of prayer, but did not feel that he was an adequate representative to be doing the praying.
>
> [Mr. Convey] was in agony. I talked to him about prayer and told him that God would help him get through this. Furthermore, I assured him that God would not forget him and would forgive a genuinely contrite heart. I gave him a copy of

the New Testament...and referred him to Philippians 4:4–7, "Rejoice in the Lord always. I shall say it again: Rejoice! Your kindness should be known to all. The Lord is near. Have no anxiety at all, but in everything, by prayer and petition, with thanksgiving, make your requests known to God. Then the peace of God that surpasses all understanding will guard your hearts and minds in Christ Jesus!"

Eileen reported that the scripture had a powerful effect on Mr. Convey, and he spoke now more positively about how he believed in the "grace of God and that God could intercede for him and his family and grant healing."

WAIT FOR THE LORD

Those who wait for the Lord shall renew their strength, they shall mount up with wings like eagles, they shall run and not be weary, they shall walk and not faint.

Isaiah 40:31

Certain translations of *Isaiah* 40:31 use the words, "They that hope in the Lord (will renew their strength") instead of "Those who wait for the Lord (will renew their strength"). The concepts of "waiting" and "hoping," however, are both understood as reflecting a posture of trust in God's ultimate care for all humankind. A commentary on the teaching notes is that, "the creator is the source of renewed power for those who are attentive to the Divine will."[10] John Collins described the meaningfulness of the passage explaining, "Hope did not come easily to the Jews during the exile. It was only possible for those who deeply believed that their God was indeed the Supreme God."[11]

Perhaps one of the hardest things for me to do is to wait. I have to confess that I'm not by nature a patient person. When I see something that needs to be done or am aware of a place I am supposed to go, my usual *modus operandi* is, "Let's get on with it! Let's not waste time! The early bird..." and so forth! My spiritual rationale for this attitude is that I believe I should be a good steward of the time God has given me and not waste precious minutes. Hmm? I wonder if that's really how God views the waiting time I so dislike?

Nurses especially, I think, do not like waiting. We've been oriented and trained to be efficient, task oriented, and to follow a hospital or health care facility schedule. That probably also makes it hard for us to encourage our patients to wait. But, so often, that's precisely what they need to do, especially during a time of recovery from illness. Just recently I told a very high-energy friend of mine who was recovering from major surgery to be "gentle" with herself, to not worry if she got tired easily, just to be patient. Sometimes we have to encourage our patients, especially our elder citizens or those facing a life-threatening illness, to be patient and to simply trust as they "wait for the Lord."

Alicia, a home care nurse, described how difficult waiting was for Mrs. Clark who "resides at home but is looked in on frequently by her sisters." Mrs. Clark "suffers from chronic inflammatory demyelinating polyneuropathy and depression; this has made her homebound." Alicia explained, Mrs. Clark "is still able to be fairly independent within the confines of home but she is at too much of a risk to her health and safety outside the home. She has suffered numerous falls while outdoors and has dropped many things in stores because of her sensory changes." Alicia recognized that caring for Mrs. Clark "would present a challenge" because as well as her "physical handicaps" she also was depressed from "waiting" in her home for the Lord to come for her or for others to come and help care for her. Alicia added, "I needed to be supportive ... she stated how hard it was for her to remain in the house but she understood that it was not safe for her to be alone in unfamiliar places."

Ultimately Alicia directed Mrs. Clark's thoughts and conversation to the positive benefits of feeding her spirit during this time of "waiting" on the Lord. Mrs. Clark admitted that her pastor came to see her every couple of weeks and that she was spiritually fulfilled with music and through programs on television. Alicia spoke with Mrs. Clark about prayer and the ways in which prayer might help her cope with her disabilities.

Often, part of the nurse's role, as with Alicia, is to help the patient focus on the good things in their lives, past and present, especially if they are in a place of "waiting" for the Lord. Reminiscences of past joys and sharing of positive present experiences can uplift a depressed elder's spirit and help the older person to focus away from illness and disability.

THE DARKNESS IS NOT DARK

Even the darkness is not dark to you; the night is as bright as the day.

Psalm 139:12

Psalm 139 is one of my favorite psalms because of its emphasis on God's interest in and care for each individual person. How comforting it is to read the psalm's opening lines that remind us that God has "searched" us and "known" us, that he even knows when we sit down or get up, he knows all our ways and can discern our thoughts from afar. Related to God's unique concern for each person, the psalmist goes on to assure the reader that wherever he or she is, the Lord's hand will be leading and thus "even the darkness will not be dark."

This psalm is sometimes described as a song "of thanksgiving in that it narrates God's merciful care...(and)...God's guidance in every part of the universe."[12]

One of the things that always amazes me is the faith and caring spirit I witness in the minds and hearts of nurses. No matter how difficult things may be in their own lives, they always seem to be able to reflect a light in the darkness to a patient's or family member's fearful experiences. I'm especially thinking of Karen, a perioperative nurse I met a few years ago when accompanying Sr. Janet, one of my Sisters who was having major surgery at a local hospital. Karen greeted us warmly in the operating room "holding area", explained the hospital's preop procedures, started Sister Janet's intravenous fluids, and helped us get Sister's operating room garb and possessions organized for the surgery.

Karen provided a sense of security in the midst of preop anxiety because of her cheerfulness and caring manner. She helped us trust that everything about the coming surgery and postoperative recovery would go well. As she proceeded through the routine preop checklist of activities, Karen chatted amiably to calm Sr. Janet's anxiety, which was noticeable. To be sociable and to also get her mind off the impending procedure, Sr. Janet began to ask Karen a few questions about her life—how long she had been working at the hospital, where she lived and so forth. We learned that Karen was a single woman who had the full responsibility of caring for her elderly mother, bedridden for the past 12 years as the result of a stroke and its sequellae.

Karen employed a health care provider to care for her mother during her own perioperative nursing shift. When she returned home after a long day at the hospital, she assumed the full nursing care responsibility for her mother. Karen relayed her story with no sense of martyrdom; it was simply what she had to do. Both Karen's care for us and her personal example provided a very bright light in the preop darkness, making that surgery morning seem not very dark at all.

IN DISTRESS YOU ARE RESCUED

I relieved your shoulder of the burden ... in distress you called and I rescued you.

Psalm 81:6–7

Psalm 81 has been described as possibly reflecting a "liturgy celebrated at one of three great festivals: Passover, Pentecost or Harvest."[13]
The Lord is thanked and celebrated for rescuing His people from distress
when He was called upon.

The psalms of David, the prayers that Jesus himself prayed, contain
wonderful messages still for us in this third millennium. Sometimes our
patients, and even ourselves as their nurses, feel that we are in distress,
that a burden has been laid on our shoulders heavier than we are able to
bear. But as Psalm 81 reminds us, if in our distress we call upon the Lord,
He will rescue us and "remove the burden from our shoulders."

Does this mean that an illness will immediately disappear, that
anxiety about a fearful diagnosis will suddenly dissipate, or that the
stress associated with our caregiving activities will be transformed into
a pink cloud of happiness? No, of course not. But what the psalmist was
reminding us was the fact that no matter what suffering we are experiencing, God is with us. He is always at our side, always ready to listen to
our prayer and to comfort us with His care and His love. And simply by
sharing our distress with the Lord in prayer, by trusting in His constant
unwavering compassion, the heaviness of our burden is, in fact, lifted
from our shoulders. Just try it and see!

I remember a time when I was hurting a great deal over a loss in my
life. After grieving for several weeks, it seemed one day that the pain was
just too much to bear. So I went into a small chapel in the residence where
I live, knelt down before the Lord, and prayed out loud (fortunately I was
alone in the chapel!): "Dear Lord, this is just too much; it's too heavy for
my shoulders. I give it to you. Please take the pain away from me."

The result was quite amazing! After my brief prayer I left the chapel, and it truly seemed that I felt an incredible sense of lightness in my
heart. Of course I was still grieving the loss but now it no longer seemed a
weighty burden; somehow I knew that I was not alone in carrying the sorrow, that my Lord and God had indeed taken the burden from my heart
and brought His presence instead. For me it was a true lived experience
of the Lord's loving care.

Frequently, we nurses have the opportunity to rescue our patients
and families in distress. Sometimes we intervene in critical situations
such as helping with a code or providing counseling for an extremely depressed patient. More often, however, we are given the daily opportunity
to "rescue" patients and families who are experiencing a variety of less
severe, but no less distressing, problems related to an illness or disability.
Laurie, a geriatric nurse, spoke about such an instance: "I was caring for
Mrs. Deaver who was a permanent resident in the nursing home because

of multiple illnesses that impacted her ability to care for herself including diabetes and a stroke incurred 3 years ago. She had right-sided weakness and needed assistance with activities of daily living. Mrs. Deaver has been homebound in the residential facility since the time of her stroke."

Laurie continued, "Mrs. Deaver admitted that she was very lonely and longed to be near family again. A cousin had recently passed away after a long battle with cancer and it turned out that this cousin ... was her last surviving relative; in her mind the last tangible connection on this earth and she had never felt so alone."

Laurie asked Mrs. Deaver if there was anything that could help her when she felt this way and the patient reached for her Bible. Together they read a portion of Psalm 25: "Look upon me, have pity on me, for I am alone and afflicted. Relieve the troubles of my heart; bring me out of distress. Put an end to my affliction and suffering."[16-18] Laurie talked with Mrs. Deaver about the strength that this passage could bring her, and they said a prayer together, reflecting on the passage. In this instance Laurie was able to help an elderly nursing home resident place the pain of her loneliness in the hands of the Lord and be reminded that she was never alone in her distress.

REJOICE IN HOPE

Rejoice in hope, be patient in suffering, persevere in prayer. Contribute to the needs of the saints; extend hospitality to strangers.

Romans 12:12–13

Chapter 12 of Saint Paul's Letter to the Romans is identified as containing the duties of the Christian community. Verses 9–12, within which is the mandate to "rejoice in hope," deal with the love that Christians should practice toward God and each other. It is suggested that the verses "appear to be a random collection of maxims, roughly rooted in the notion of disinterested love, agape."[14] Biblical scholar John Pilch notes that, "Paul's remarks all support honorable living. Above all, he says serve the Lord, do the honorable thing. Have confidence reaching out for your future (rejoice in hope)."[15] Paul is encouraging his early Roman Christian community to practice faith-filled hope and trust in God.

When we look at the mandates of the above scripture quotation, it seems somewhat incongruous that the Lord should ask us to rejoice while we are also trying to be patient in suffering. I believe that most of us, and most of our patients, find it difficult to be "patient" in suffering, much less to be joyful while experiencing some painful sorrow.

But, of course, Saint Paul's emphasis here, the call to be joyful, is associated with the virtue of hope, not the concept of sorrow. Hope is not, however, always an easy virtue to embrace, especially in times of suffering. This is particularly true for the Irish. At least, that's what an Irish missionary sister friend once told me. Sister Mary Ellen said that the Irish are great in practicing faith and charity but hope, we're not so good at. I remember once reading something to the effect that only an Irishman (or woman, of course) could arise on a beautiful sunny spring morning to the chirping of birds and the feel of balmy delicious weather without a cloud in the sky and immediately think, "Well, it'll probably be raining buckets by the end of the day"! We Irish do not usually tend to "look on the bright side." I have, in the past, quipped that perhaps we've never recovered from the potato famine! But, looking at it more seriously, perhaps a fear of famine was so deeply instilled into our culture during those truly dark days in Irish history that we really do fear becoming complacent even when things seem to be going well.

And, one doesn't need to be Irish to have similar fears. A variety of painful past life experiences with such situations as family need, work-related problems, financial difficulties, or a host of other stressors can make hope elusive, especially for one dealing with a serious acute or chronic illness or injury. It is, nevertheless, especially in times of illness or disability that we most need to embrace such virtues as hope, patience, and prayer.

Not all of our patients are able to find joy in hope; sometimes it's just a kind of "hanging on with one's fingernails," so to speak, but a person may still have a sense of hope even in the midst of anxiety. For others the hope is a source of joy. Mary, a surgical nurse, told of one such patient, "I was working on an orthopedic floor and caring for Rita, a 19-year-old girl. She had been in a serious car accident and needed a series of surgeries to repair her injuries. She was a great reminder to me of how little it takes to show someone you care, to be a sign of God's hope to that patient."

Mary reported that Rita kept an "upbeat attitude" but "expressed a need to have her appearance tended to. She just hated looking as though she had been confined to a hospital bed. I had forgotten how important that was at her age.... She needed someone to do the trivial things not really important to her care but extremely important to her recovery! Things that allowed her to keep her positive attitude, her hope, and promote her healing."

Mary continued, "All she needed was someone to wash her hair and get her a new pair of socks for her unaffected leg. I got another nurse to help me and we created the "(Hospital) Hair Salon." This may have seemed almost silly but it was so important to this young woman; she got washed and styled and looked great."

Mary concluded, "I cannot even describe the immense gratitude that Rita had; she just needed to feel loved and cared for!"

This chapter is about ways a patient may be encouraged to find peace, hope, and even a sense of joy in the midst of suffering. Nurses in their spiritual ministry of caring may, at times, have the opportunity to guide and support their chronically or seriously ill patients in trusting in the compassionate and tender caring of the Lord who wishes only good for humankind. The challenges to such faith can be immense, especially for a younger person dealing with a terminal or life-threatening illness or for the parents of a dying child. And the challenges to a nurse ministering in such situations can also be immense. Thus nurses as well as their patients must always remember that ultimately faith in the resurrected Lord has been promised to bring about for all believers the ending of "winter."

A NURSE'S PRAYER FOR FAITHFULNESS

The fruit of the spirit is love, joy, peace, patience, kindness, faithfulness, gentleness and self-control.

Galatians 5:22

O Holy Spirit, who inspires and guides each step of my nursing ministry, bless me with the gift of faithfulness. When things seem darkest, help me to trust in Your light; when things seem harshest, help me to trust in Your gentleness; when things seem frustrating, help me to trust in Your peace; and when everything seems to be falling apart, help me to have faith. Let me never forget that You are always with me, loving, protecting, caring, and supporting. Let me always remain faithful to my nursing ministry of caring. Teach me, Dear Holy Spirit, to be a vessel of Your love for all for whom I care. Amen.

8   A Deserted Place: The Mysticism of Everyday Nursing

In the morning, while it was still dark, he got up and went out to a deserted place, and there he prayed.

Mark 1:35

A HIDDEN MINISTRY

Gentle Jesus, you who lived for many
years a life of hidden ministry,
teach Your nurses to live the
hidden ministry of our
discipleship:

the hidden ministry of solicitously
feeding a hungry elder;

the hidden ministry of caringly
giving water to a thirsty child;

the hidden ministry of kindly
welcoming a stranger to
hospital admission;

the hidden ministry of comfortingly
putting a warm blanket on a
chilled patient;

the hidden ministry of mercifully
visiting a sister or brother

> *imprisoned in a nursing*
>   *home;*
>
> *the hidden ministry of supportively*
>   *counseling a newly diagnosed*
>   *cancer patient;*
>
> *the hidden ministry of sitting compassionately*
>   *at the bedside of one*
>   *who is dying.*
>
> *Help Your nurses to remember, Dear Lord,*
>   *that in these, the hidden ministries,*
>   *we care not only for our patients,*
>   *we care also for You!*

It seems appropriate for this final chapter of a book about the spiritual ministry of nursing to focus on the nurse's personal spirituality, on the quiet times when he or she can, as Jesus, go away to "a deserted place" to meditate and pray. Finding such "quiet time" is not easy for those of us who are daily in the midst of the "madding crowds" in such settings as the hospital unit, the clinic, the physician's office, patients' homes, schools, churches, or the university. Somehow it seems for nurses there is always work to be done: patient needs to be met, care plans to be completed, or management issues to be dealt with. The idea of quiet time may seem very far-fetched indeed as we look at our jammed daily or weekly calendar of activities.

But, quiet time may have seemed far-fetched to Jesus also. Surely the Divine Son of God knew that His earthly ministry was limited, at least limited according to human time. And yet we are told by the evangelist Mark that Jesus took the time to go away to a deserted place to pray. Is our work, our ministry of nursing, more important than the ministry of the Lord?

Scripture scholars commenting on the passage recorded in *Mark* 1:35 offer several takes on the meaning of Jesus withdrawing to a deserted place to pray. Van Linden asserts that Jesus "withdraws to a desert place to pray alone because he knows that people are seeking him out only because of his miraculous powers. They have misunderstood him," Van Linden adds, "and so he must move on to neighboring villages and continue his ministry of preaching and healing throughout all of Galilee."[1] This thought is supported by Paul Achtemeier who noted that although "crowds were clamoring" for Jesus, he "chose to withdraw, first for prayer, and then to go to other regions. He had been sent to announce the nearness of God's final rule, and success or even human need, could not deter him from spreading that announcement."[2] Hahn and Mitch observe, additionally, that *Mark* 1:35 reveals that "Jesus practices what he preaches on the propriety of solitary prayer."[3]

So what do these interpretations have to say to us as nurses? In the ministry that we have been called by God to embrace, this living out of a sacred covenant with those for whom we care, do we also not need to periodically refresh our spirits? Do we not need to "withdraw to a deserted place" to reclaim in our hearts the true meaning of Jesus teaching of our nursing, "Truly, I tell you, just as you did it to one of the least of these who are members of my family, you did it to me" (*Matthew* 25:40)? Do we not, as Jesus Himself recognized, need to prepare ourselves through solitary prayer and meditation to continue spreading the announcement of God's love through our ministry of nursing to the next fearful patient we meet, to the next anxious family, to the next dying elder?

Although remaining committed to our calling, we must not become so captive to compulsive "busyness" that our ministry of caring is injured by the intrusion of such spiritual maladies as apathy and frustration. We must provide for ourselves the spiritual "medicine" necessary to keep alive the joy and the peace and the satisfaction experienced in the blessed ministry of caring for our ill brothers and sisters. We are truly graced to have been called to a ministry that Jesus Himself blessed with His mandate to serve; we must always treasure and protect the gift.

THIRSTING FOR GOD

As a deer longs for flowing streams, so my soul longs for you, O God. My soul thirsts for God, for the living God.

Psalm 42:1–2

In commenting on Psalm 42, biblical scholar Richard Clifford suggests that the song is one of "lament of an individual...who longs to join the community of God."[4] "What distresses the psalmist," Clifford notes, "is the absence of God, the feeling of deep hunger without the ability to satisfy it because of distance from Jerusalem and the hindrance of enemies."[5] And, don't we nurses sometimes feel that hunger for God, a hunger sometimes caused by a distancing from Him brought about by enemies hidden within the demands of our work?

As I ponder this scripture, I can't help but think of times in my life when I have become so immersed in my nursing activities that I had minimal time for prayer and meditation. This is a condition that I've named "spiritual malnutrition." One can manage to live on the "junk food" of an occasional quick prayer for a while, but ultimately the spirit cries out with yearning for the "living waters" of a true relationship with God.

Sometimes our work schedules really do hinder our spiritual needs, but hopefully this will not become a consistent pattern. A rather dramatic personal incident comes to mind from many years ago. I had always looked forward to Midnight Mass on Christmas Eve. One year, in my early nursing career, I was forced to spend an entire Christmas holiday working evenings at a small rural hospital to help finance completion of a college degree. The hospital was about an hour's drive on country roads from the school dorm where I had been allowed to remain over the Christmas break. The Sisters who ran the college told me they had planned a beautiful Christmas Eve liturgy and invited me to participate. They would leave a door unlocked for me to join them as soon as I got home from work. I hastened through the 3–11 end-of-shift report, jumped into my car, and hit the road for home as fast as I dared drive on the icy highway. I arrived back at the college delighted that I had a good 5 minutes to spare and would not be late for the service. I rushed to the building housing our chapel only to find that the door, which was supposed to be left open, had accidentally been locked. As there were several entrances to the building, I ran hopefully from one door to the other only to find everything locked up tight. I could see lights illuminating the beautiful stained glass chapel windows and hear the Christmas music emanating from the organ, but there simply was no way in.

Finally, in desperation I trudged back to my car and headed off to a local church, about 20 minutes away. Obviously, I arrived quite late, did not know anyone in the crowded congregation, had to stand in the back of the church, and missed a great deal of the service. I can still remember my tears that evening because I wanted so much to be present for a joyful Christmas Eve celebration of the Lord's birthday. I might have used my experience to meditate on Our Lady's finding no place in Bethlehem's Inn if I had been holier. I'm afraid, however, that all I could feel was disappointed and lonely on that Christmas Eve, as well as a deep yearning for the spiritual experience I had anticipated.

A positive benefit of my being "locked out" that Christmas Eve, however, was the recognition that as much as I love nursing and loved my holiday evenings at the small rural hospital, I also desired time to be with the Lord, to pray and to refresh my spirit so that I would receive the strength and the grace to be able to bring His love to my patients and their families. I pray that all of us, as nurses, never lose our "thirst" for a true and meaningful relationship with the "living God."

THE DESERT OF YOUR HEART

He sustained him in a desert land, in a howling wilderness waste;
he shielded him, cared for him, guarded him as the apple of his eye.

Deuteronomy 32:10

The Old Testament Book of Deuteronomy is identified as "a series of sermons given by Moses;"[6] the sermons are described as Moses' teachings to his people.[7] Chapter 32, entitled *The Song of Moses*, contained Moses' proclamation of the greatness, the perfection, and the justice of God. In the epic song, Moses related how a faithful God cared for His people even when they had "dealt falsely with him." Moses described how God "sustained (Jacob) in a desert land, in a howling wilderness waste; he shielded him, cared for him, guarded him as the apple of his eye" and added a metaphor for emphasis: "As an eagle stirs up its nest, and hovers over its young; as it spreads its wings, takes them up, and bears them aloft on its pinions, the Lord alone guided him."

As in the Gospel of Mark cited earlier (1:35), the concept of desert emerges in the Deuteronomy scripture, this time highlighting a solitary place where God protects and cares for His people. I've never lived in the desert personally but have known some Sisters who have. They speak both of its awesome beauty and frightful isolation, of its enervating heat during the day and bone-chilling cold at night. The desert is a place where one can commune deeply with God yet be totally isolated from other people. Those who have spent time in the desert affirm that it changes one, always for the better.

But how can we as busy, committed, professional nurses manage to spend time in the desert to grow closer to the Lord, to understand ourselves more completely and to listen for His voice? In writing about prayer, the gentle Francis de Sales taught that busy people could encounter the desert by periodically withdrawing into themselves. Francis advised, "Retire at various times into the deserts of your own heart even while outwardly engaged in discussions or engagements with others. The mental retreat cannot be penetrated by the people around you. They are standing around your body, not your heart. Your heart remains in the presence of God alone."[8]

The message of Francis de Sales is echoed also in the writing of Carmelite Brother Lawrence of the Resurrection who asserted, "It is not necessary for being with God to be always at church. We may make an oratory of our heart wherein to retire from time to time to converse with him in meekness, humility and love."[9] The concept is reinforced by the words of Brother Roger of Taize who noted, "In each person there is a portion of solitude which no human intimacy can ever fill. Yet, you are never alone...in your heart of hearts, in the place where no two people are alike, Christ is waiting for you."[10]

When we nurses attempt to live the messages of Francis de Sales, Brother Lawrence, and Brother Roger in the midst of our busy days, when we try from "time to time" to "retire" to the desert of our heart, we will receive the strength and the courage needed for our spiritual ministry of caring.

An anecdote related by a new graduate nurse, Vicki, reflects the beauty of such caring that she perceived in a nursing ministry to her dying aunt:

> My aunt had stomach cancer. Her tumor was so large that it was not logical to operate on it; in addition to the stomach cancer, she had already developed metastasis to her liver.... [After the physician told her the diagnosis] she had a look of shock, disbelief, and dismay on her face. She was a strong, independent, extremely successful woman that I had never seen even remotely close to tears in my life, suddenly reduced to a puddle of emotion.... I gave her a large hug; she thought that I was consoling her but my heart needed the embrace as well. Suddenly, I realized that I did not care if the hospital bed corners were perfectly tucked or if her bed was angled at 30 degrees, I cared about my aunt, about her life, and the quality she would have for the remainder of it.
>
> My aunt was transferred to the oncology unit and asked me to stay with her that evening; we were writing out Christmas cards that she wanted to send, even if she didn't survive until December, when suddenly there was a knock on the door and an evening nurse, Sheila, entered the room. I was baffled; it wasn't time for a meal, treatment, or medications. What could she possibly need or want? I sat quietly in the corner reading a book and to my delight, Sheila held my aunt's hand and consoled her.
>
> Sheila didn't dwell on my aunt's disease but rather just talked to her, discovering her interests and talents. Sheila was celebrating my aunt's life, making her feel good about all she had done and not dwelling on her infirmity. She rubbed her

back and helped her relax and I could sense and see peace within my aunt. Sheila stayed for only 30 minutes but it felt like 3 hours. My aunt and I finished her cards and she asked me to hold her hand as she fell asleep.

Vicki ended her story: "My aunt passed from this world 2 days later. Through it all I remembered Sheila's compassion and caring demeanor. She took the time to listen to my aunt, to care.... Sheila provided an example for me that I hope I never forget and a model of all that I hope to emulate in my own nursing career." I believe that it was Sheila's own faith and ability to "retire" at times to the "desert" of her heart that allowed her to truly be the loving, caring, needed presence for Vicki's aunt in her last hours.

IN HIS PRESENCE

You have upheld me...and set me in your presence forever.

Psalm 41:13

Psalm 41, a psalm of David, is described as "a psalm of thanksgiving" that "recounts God's rescue of a sick individual...recovery from illness is a mark of favor showing God's love for this individual."[11] The psalmist extols God's loving care for His people who become ill: "The Lord sustains them on their sickbed; in their illness you heal all their infirmities" (41:3). The psalmist adds in praising God, "You have upheld me...and set me in your presence forever" (41:13).

Much has been written about the presence of God, especially the practice of the presence of God. Brother Lawrence of the Resurrection, author of *The Practice of the Presence of God,* advised, "We do not have to be constantly in church to be with God. We can make our heart a prayer room into which we can retire from time to time to converse with Him, gently, humbly, lovingly. Everyone is capable of these familiar conversations with God."[12] Spiritual writer Wayne Simsic uses the expression "mindfulness" to reflect our practice of God's presence: "Through attention to our daily activities, we awaken to the presence of God in the moment and discover that our life is prayer.... Mindfulness, then, is not an exercise in concentration but a posture of heart, an attitude of trust in God's presence within every activity."[13]

In the previous pages Sheila revealed her practice of presence to a suffering patient; in essence Sheila's presence to Vicki's aunt was also a presence to the God who dwells within her heart. This concept is reflected in the Hindu greeting *Namaste,* a formal definition of which relates to a salutation to a person's inner self but which many people understand as meaning, "the God living within me greets the God living within you."

Nurse Jan Pettigrew identified five distinguishing features of "presence": self-giving to the other person at the moment at hand, being available and at the disposal of the other person with all of self for that period of time, listening with a tangible awareness of the privilege one has in being allowed to participate in such an experience, listening in a way that involves giving of oneself, and being there in a way that the other person defines as meaningful.[14] Pettigrew's attributes of presence read as the definition of a caring nurse–patient interaction. When we practice the presence of God in our nursing ministry, caregiving activities will, in fact, be characterized by self-giving by turning our minds and hearts away from personal concerns to those of our patient; being available by somehow managing to find the time to be totally focused on an ill person's needs and how they might be met; listening…(with) awareness of privilege, that is, lovingly and caringly listening, as Saint Benedict so poignantly put it, "with the ear of the heart"; listening…giving of oneself by listening with the real desire to respond to whatever pain or worry is shared; and being there in a way the other person defines as meaningful by being so completely attuned to the presence of the sick person or a family member that he or she knows, without doubt, that the nurse's caring presence is complete, unwavering, and totally committed to promoting the well-being of another. This latter posture of presence can be reflected not only in a nurse's words but also in posture, in eye contact, and in a gentle and nonjudgmental attitude.

A HIDDEN MINISTRY

There is nothing hidden, except to be disclosed; nor in anything secret, except to come to light.

Mark 4:22

The scripture quotation above is taken from Jesus' "Parable of the Lamp": "(Jesus) said to them, 'Is a lamp brought in to be put under the bushel basket or under the bed, and not on the lampstand? For there is nothing hidden except to be disclosed; nor in anything secret except to come to light. Let anyone with ears to hear listen!'" (*Mark* 4:21–23). This scripture passage is frequently thought to mean that one should not hide talents (light) under a bushel but should share them with the world (placing them on a lampstand instead of in hiding). Scripture scholar Van Linden notes that "by the parable of the lamp, Mark suggests that his readers will have to ponder the meaning of Jesus' life and message much more thoroughly for themselves before they can share it fully with others";[15] and Paul Achtemeier points out that the Greek of the verse actually reads, "Does a lamp come in order to be put under a bushel or under a bed? But what 'lamp' is thus able to 'come'? Clearly it refers to Jesus. Though the light of the kingdom he brings now seems dim or even hidden, it will, yet, in its time, become manifest."[16]

Matthew's recording of the parable includes a specific mandate from Jesus to his disciples: "You are the light of the world. A city built on a hill cannot be hid. No one after lighting a lamp puts it under the bushel basket, but on the lampstand, and it gives light to all in the house. In the same way, let your light shine before others, so that they may see your good works and give glory to your father in heaven" (5:14–16). Daniel Harrington, in commenting on Matthew's text of the "Parable of the Lamp," interprets the meaning as related specifically to the ministry of Jesus' disciples whom, Matthew notes, he called "the light of the world" (*Matthew* 5:14): "When Jesus calls his disciples the light of the world, he says that their actions serve as a beacon of light in a dark world. The disciples are challenged to let their light shine as a witness to their fidelity to Jesus and his heavenly father."[17]

We, as nurses, are also challenged to "let our light shine," but because of the nature of our caregiving activities, frequently our "light" is restricted to each individual patient or family interaction in which we participate. Often the caring activities, so appreciated by patients and families, are not reported, not charted, and many times not even spoken about with coworkers. Thus I have labeled nursing as a "hidden" ministry, as I have also, as noted earlier, labeled nurses as "anonymous ministers."

In a study entitled, "The Nurse, the Anonymous Minister," which explored spiritual care as carried out by a group of 66 practicing nurses, the concept of the nurse's hidden ministry was described as "non-verbalized theology."[18] The conceptual label "non-verbalized theology" was identified by one of the study participants, Paula, a doctorally prepared medical-surgical nurse with 22 years of experience. Paula observed, "Ministry is not a discreet function: a separate task. It is embedded in the careful giving of the meds, the wiping of the brow, the asking of the right questions, the acknowledgment of the patient's humanness, and what they are experiencing in their sickness. I can be there to be a person of the love of God. You want to alleviate suffering, convey hope, bring love. It is in giving your care in a caring way, but there is no theology being verbalized; it's a non-verbalized theology."[19]

A brief, yet powerful, nurse–patient interaction that illustrates the "hidden ministry" is that of Joanne's care for Mrs. Jones. Joanne stopped in Mrs. Jones' room to check on her; Mrs. Jones was a woman in her late seventies battling breast cancer. Joanne explained:

> In addition to her cancer [Mrs. Jones] lost her sight to cataracts some years ago, and for this reason must be looked after by caregivers.... [Mrs. Jones] was quite anxious on the day of our first meeting but on this, the day of our second, she seemed downright apprehensive about something. In talking to her she disclosed that she had an appointment with her physician later on in the afternoon to reveal the results of a PET scan to determine if her disease had spread. She was quite beside herself and apologized repeatedly for how disheveled and discombobulated she was. She said she did not know if there was a lot of point in talking to me; she just felt she could not focus.

Joanne told Mrs. Jones that she understood and added, "I just asked that we might pray together before I left. We prayed for her and we prayed for her doctors and caregivers." Joanne reported that she then shared a scripture passage about God's care and support with Mrs. Jones and it brought her consolation. Joanne concluded, "It was one of the shortest [patient] interactions I have ever had, and one of the simplest verses of scripture, but it was so profound!"

Probably no one except Joanne and Mrs. Jones, and now I with whom Joanne shared her experience, knew about this powerful nursing ministry of caring, a ministry of light but yet, for all intents and purposes, a "hidden ministry."

THE MYSTICISM OF EVERYDAY NURSING

Now we see in a mirror, dimly, but then we will see face to face.
Now I know only in part; then I will know fully, even as I have
been fully known. And now faith, hope, and love abide, these three;
and the greatest of these is love.

1 Corinthians 13:12–13

The scripture passage above contains a message that might be considered to be the central theme of nursing practice, that of the predominance of love above all other virtues. The entire passage, from Paul's first letter to the Corinthian community, is entitled "The Gift of Love." Paul's message begins with the admonition, "If I speak in tongues…but do not have love, I am a noisy gong or a clanging cymbal. And, if I have prophetic powers…and all knowledge…and all faith…but do not have love, I am nothing. If I give away all my possessions...but do not have love, I gain nothing" (13:1-3). Paul continues on with the classic definition of love, "Love is patient; love is kind; love is not envious or boastful or arrogant or rude. It does not insist on its own way; it is not irritable or resentful; it does not rejoice in wrongdoing, but rejoices in the truth. It bears all things, believes all things, hopes all things, endures all things. Love never ends" (13:4-8).

As cited above, Paul ends the well-known teaching by reminding the young Christian community that such things as prophecies and knowledge will come to an end as they are only partial and not complete attributes; now we think as "children" but ultimately we will reason as "adults." Thus, Paul concludes, "For now we see in a mirror, dimly, but then we will see face to face. Now I know only in part; then I will know fully, even as I have been fully known. And now faith, hope and love abide, these three; and the greatest of these is love" (13:12-13).

Biblical scholar Mary Ann Getty, in commenting on the above passage of Paul's letter, notes, "Love is the more excellent way. In understanding this very famous passage, we need to bear in mind Paul's description of charity as the gift of the community. It is the more excellent way, which is also the more fundamental way, the way for all."[20] Getty underscores the fact that Paul was admonishing the Corinthians that they were thinking as children because he wanted the community to realize that "even the clearest knowledge is like a shadow compared to love," that as they grow they will realize that "only love lasts."[21]

I can't help but think how appropriate these words of Saint Paul, penned so many centuries ago, are for we 21st century nurses. Much is written, currently, about the importance of the professionalization of nursing, about research and scholarly productivity, especially for those of us in the academic world. Such professional attributes are also identified for practitioners of nursing as many hospitals seek to elect the prestigious designation of "Magnet Status." This is positive, of course, as nursing must always strive to keep step with changes and advances in medicine and health care overall.

When, however, one reflects on the myriad, real-world, third millennium stories of nurse–patient interactions shared in the preceding pages, it is indeed the nurse's *love* for his or her patients and families and for the practice of nursing that is so deeply appreciated by those who are ill and their loved ones. It is the nurse's *love* that undergirds not only the skilled care provided to those in need but also the *kindness* with which that care is given. It is the nurse's *love* that supports the ability to be *patient* with the ill who are angry or hurt because of their suffering. It is the nurse's *love* that prevents him or her from becoming *arrogant* or *rude* when patients or families demand the impossible because of their anxieties and fears about the course of an injury or illness. It is *love* that allows a nurse to be flexible in meeting patients' needs, not insisting that everything be done his or her *own way*; it is nurses' *love* that prevents them from becoming *irritable* or *resentful* even when caregiving requests seem demanding beyond reason. The nurse's *love* discourages *wrongdoing* in the practice of caring and emphasizes *truth* in all patient interactions. And, finally, especially on those difficult days when the treasured practice of one's profession may seem, in the moment, more like a burden than a gift, it is the nurses' *love* of their blessed calling to minister to the ill and the injured that *bears all things, believes all things, hopes all things* and *endures all things*.

Related to the nurse's love, shared in the patient care anecdotes of all of the previous chapters, it is not inappropriate to label "everyday nursing" as containing a dimension of mysticism. Over and over the nurse's stories of patient and family interactions reflect amazing instances of caring behaviors on the part of nurses. Simple not unusual activities such as holding a patient's hand, listening to a patient's pain, treating a patient and/or family with respect and kindness, or sharing a brief prayer brought about both healing and deep gratitude on the part of the care recipients. This is truly the mysticism of everyday nursing.

Historically, the term mysticism has been "understood in radically different ways."[22] One way of defining the concept is as "a loving knowledge of God which is born in a personal encounter with the divine."[23] Brother Roger of Taize, speaking of mystical contemplation, observed that it was "quite simply the attitude in which our whole being is totally seized by the wonder of a presence.... It is the whole of our being, emotions and all, that is seized by the reality of the love of God."[24] Thelma Hall describes the contemplative prayer of a mystic as the result of "being literally 'in love' with God, at the deepest level of the relationship with him for which we are created."[25]

Spiritual writer Stephen Hatch asserts that "everyone has the potential to become a fully transformed mystic."[26] Hatch's belief supports my earlier conceptualization of the "mysticism of everyday nursing" published in *Spirituality in Nursing, Standing on Holy Ground*.[27] The concept of nursing mysticism is also derived from the writings of theologian Karl Rahner who contended that "everyone is at least an anonymous mystic."[28] Rahner believed that "wherever there is radical self-forgetting for the sake of the other...there is...the mysticism of everyday life."[29]

Florence Nightingale's understanding of mysticism among nurses has been described as "practical mysticism," which refers to "the experience of a mystic—someone whose direct experience of God and the divine reveals the presence of the divine everywhere — whose sense of spirituality and action are so mutual and integrated as to be impossible to distinguish the two."[30] Nightingale also wrote that what she meant by mystical theology was "what Christ meant. He was the first great mystic who was at once yet the most active reformer that ever lived."[31]

Florence's writings on theology continued a practical approach to mysticism; she observed, "It appears to me that the mystical state is the essence of common sense if it is real, that is, if God is a reality. We can only act and speak and think through him and the thing is to discover such laws of his as will enable us to be always acting and thinking in conscious concert of cooperation with him."[32] Nightingale asserted, "This is the true mystical doctrine: where shall I find God? In myself. But then I myself must be in a state for him to come and dwell in me."[33]

As suggested earlier, many 21st century nurses are indeed the practical mystics that our founder Florence Nightingale envisioned. A geriatric nurse who beautifully exemplifies nursing as a mystical ministry to which she has been called by God is Suzanne.

Suzanne described the importance of the hidden ministry of simple caring nursing tasks in her interactions with two patients, Miss Gorden and Mr. Connors. Miss Gorden was an elderly Parkinson's disease patient that she had cared for: "I can't help but recall how Miss Gorden's face lit up when I offered to help her eat. She did not see it as pointing to her disability but as caring enough to stop my other duties to help her. I then helped her brush her hair, which looked as though it hadn't been touched in days. I feel that those are the simple things we are called to do, just as *Matthew* 25:35–37 calls us to do when we care for the brothers and sisters who are suffering."

Mr. Connors was a frail octogenarian, with multiple diagnoses, residing in a nursing home. Suzanne explained, "We had several lively chats. We talked about many things from the NBA basketball season to politics, but mostly about matters of faith. He often talked about how he was afraid of death and afraid of becoming ill with some disease because he did not know what he would do. At one point I saw this elderly, free-spirited, whimsical man practically crumbling before me." Suzanne continued, "I asked [Mr. Connors] if he wanted to pray with me. He agreed. We sat silently, with our eyes closed, just holding each other's hands." Suzanne then shared a biblical passage describing God's love and support that was very comforting to Mr. Connors. She concluded, "God led me to that particular passage, and it was what he needed to hear."

This chapter has presented myriad nursing anecdotes reflecting the mysticism of everyday nursing. There are stories of practical mysticism, as envisioned by Florence Nightingale in the 19th century and now carried out by contemporary nurses in the third millennium. The patient interaction anecdotes reflect not only nurses' dedication and caring but also strong faith and trust in their calling to serve in ministry to the ill and the injured. Nurses of the 21st century do indeed embrace and live the mysticism of everyday nursing.

In an earlier book, *Spirituality in Nursing: Standing on Holy Ground,*[34] I explored spirituality in nursing focusing on such topics as a nursing theology of caring, a spiritual history of nursing, nursing assessment of patients' spiritual needs, the nurse's role in spiritual care, and the spiritual needs of diverse groups of patients and family members amenable to nursing intervention. These patient populations included those who were acutely ill, those who were chronically ill, children and families, older adults, the terminally ill (end of life, death and bereavement), and persons involved in mass casualty disasters.

The present work has been written as an extension of and companion to *Spirituality in Nursing.* In *A Sacred Covenant* key themes focused on the nurse' covenant with a patient, the nurse as minister, the nurse's tradition of service, the nurse's compassion, the nurse's devotion and commitment to caring, the nurse's vulnerability, and the nurse's faith. All these concepts, which emerged from both clinical experience and discussions with practicing nurses, unequivocally led to the conclusion that "everyday nursing" did indeed contain an element of mysticism, the undergirding theme of the final chapter.

This is not an easy time to be a nurse. Many hospitals and clinics are understaffed, patient care has become more complex than in any past health care era, and financial issues often drive the kind and degree of treatment that a patient receives.

This is also a blessed time to be a nurse. The challenges are great but nurses have, for centuries, been challenged to greatness. We have only to look at our nursing forebears for inspiration. Writing from the Crimea in 1854, Florence Nightingale admitted, "I have not a moment. The whole army is coming into the hospitals. The task will be gigantic. Alas, how will it end? We are in the hands of God. Pray for us. We have at the moment five thousand sick and wounded. My only comfort is, God sees it, God knows it, God loves us."[35]

As our foundress so poignantly observed, "God sees" our nursing challenges, "God knows" our nursing challenges, "God loves us." How blessed we are, as 21st century nurses, to be called as Florence Nightingale to a ministry of caring that God sees, God knows, and, truly, God loves.

A NURSE'S PRAYER IN HIDDENNESS

Indeed, the word of God is living and active . . . it is able to judge the thoughts and intentions of the heart. And before him no (one) is hidden.

Hebrews 4:12–13

Gentle God, I thank You for my nursing ministry of hiddenness. I thank You for my hidden ministry of feeding a hungry child, for my hidden ministry of giving a drink of water to a thirsty accident victim, for my hidden ministry of putting a warm blanket on a chilled post-op patient, for my hidden ministry of welcoming a new patient to the hospital, for my hidden ministry of visiting an elder imprisoned in a nursing home, and for my hidden ministry of carrying out the myriad daily activities of caring for the sick.

I thank You for the hiddenness of my nursing that is seen only by You, O Lord of my life and Master of my heart. Grant me the grace to always remember that in the hiddenness of the ministry of nursing lies the treasure of becoming Your disciple. I thank You for calling me to follow You in this most blessed and hidden ministry. Amen.

References

CHAPTER 1: A SACRED COVENANT: The Spiritual Ministry of Nursing

1. Henri Nouwen, *Creative Ministry* (New York: Image Books, 1991), 56.
2. David Alexander and Pat Alexander, eds., *Eerdmans Handbook to the Bible* (Grand Rapids, MI: Wm. B. Eerdmans Publishing Co., 1992), 134.
3. Ibid.
4. Jerome H. Neyrey, *First Timothy, Second Timothy, Titus, James, First Peter, Second Peter, Jude* (Collegeville, MN: The Liturgical Press, 1986), 28.
5. Ibid.
6. M. Patricia Donahue, *Nursing, the Finest Art,* 2nd edition (St. Louis, MO: Mosby, 1996), 75.
7. Ibid.
8. Ibid.
9. Lavinia L. Dock and Isabel M. Stewart, *A Short History of Nursing: From the Earliest Times to the Present Day* (New York: G.P. Putnam's Sons, 1920), 42.
10. Ibid.
11. Ibid.
12. Barbara M. Dossey, *Florence Nightingale: Mystic, Visionary, Healer* (Springhouse, PA: Springhouse Publications, 2000), 3.
13. Victor Robinson, *White Caps: The Story of Nursing* (Philadelphia: J.B. Lippincott Company, 1946), 126.
14. Ibid., 127.
15. John J. Collins, *Isaiah* (Collegeville, MN: The Liturgical Press, 1986), 94.
16. Kenneth Baker, *Inside the Bible: An Introduction to Each Book of the Bible* (San Francisco: Ignatius Press, 1998), 149.
17. Neyrey, 77.
18. Joyce Rupp, *May I Have This Dance?* (Notre Dame, IN: Ave Maria Press, 1992), 117.
19. Ibid.
20. Caryll Houselander, *The Reed of God* (Allen, TX: Christian Classics, 1978), 1.
21. Ibid.
22. Ibid., 8.
23. Ibid.

24. Ann D. Kilmer and Daniel A. Foxvog, "Music," in *Harper's Bible Dictionary,* ed. Paul J. Achtemeier (New York: Harper & Row, 1985), 670.

25. Mary Elizabeth O'Brien, *Prayer in Nursing: The Spirituality of Compassionate Caregiving* (Sudbury, MA: Jones and Bartlett Publishers, 2003), 57–59.

26. Mary Elizabeth O'Brien, *Spirituality in Nursing: Standing on Holy Ground,* 2nd edition (Sudbury, MA: Jones and Bartlett Publishers, 2003), 84–86.

27. Mary Elizabeth O'Brien, *The Nurse With an Alabaster Jar: A Biblical Approach to Nursing* (Madison, WI: NCF Press, 2006), 95–100.

CHAPTER 2: MINISTERS OF A NEW COVENANT: The Spirituality of Caregiving

1.   Jane Hudson, *How to Become a Trained Nurse* (New York: William Abbatt, 1897), 14.

2.   Mary Ann Getty, *First Corinthians, Second Corinthians* (Collegeville, MN: The Liturgical Press, 1991), 95.

3.   Jerome Kodell, *The Gospel According to Luke* (Collegeville, MN: The Liturgical Press, 1989), 33–34.

4.   George W. MacRae and Daniel J. Harrington, "Invitation to John," in *Invitation to the Gospels,* eds. Paul J. Achtemeier, Daniel J. Harrington, Robert J. Karris, George W. MacRae, and Donald Senior (Mahwah, NJ: Paulist Press, 2002), 325–405.

5.   Neal M. Flanagan, *The Gospel According to John and the Johannine Epistles* (Collegeville, MN: The Liturgical Press, 1989), 19.

6.   Barbara M. Dossey, *Florence Nightingale: Mystic, Visionary, Healer* (Springhouse, PA: Springhouse Corporation, 2000), 33.

7.   Kodell, 31.

8.   Cornelius J. van der Poel, "Health Care Ministry: A Human and Christian Task," in *Wholeness and Holiness: A Christian Response to Suffering,* ed. C.J. van der Poel (Franklin, WI: Sheed & Ward, 1999), 1–14.

9.   Daniel J. Harrington, *The Gospel According to Matthew* (Collegeville, MN: The Liturgical Press, 1991), 78.

10. Donald Senior, "Invitation to Matthew," in *Invitation to the Gospels* (Mahwah, NJ: Paulist Press, 2002), 71.

11. Mary Elizabeth O'Brien, *Spirituality in Nursing: Standing on Holy Ground,* 2nd edition (Sudbury, MA: Jones and Bartlett Publishers, 2003).

12. Senior, 91.

13. Scott Hahn and Curtis Mitch, *The Gospel of Matthew* (San Francisco: Ignatius Press, 2000), 64.

CHAPTER 3: VARIETIES OF GIFTS: A Tradition of Service

1. Mary Ann Getty, *First Corinthians, Second Corinthians* (Collegeville, MN: The Liturgical Press, 1991), 54.

2. Donald Senior, "Invitation to Matthew," in *Invitation to the Gospels*, eds. Donald Senior, Paul J. Achtemeier, Robert J. Karras, George W. MacRae, and Daniel J. Harrington (Mahwah, NJ: Paulist Press, 2002), 1–106.

3. Ben C. Johnson, *Pastoral Spirituality: A Focus for Ministry* (Philadelphia: The Westminister Press, 1988), 133.

4. Barbara M. Dossey, *Florence Nightingale: Mystic, Visionary, Healer* (Springhouse, PA: Springhouse Corporation, 2000), 33.

5. Florence Nightingale, *Notes on Nursing: What It Is and What It Is Not* (London: Harrison, 1859), 71.

6. Margaret Baly, ed., *As Miss Nightingale Said...Florence Nightingale Through Her Sayings: A Victorian Perspective* (London: Scutari Press, 1991), 68.

7. Isabel Hampton Robb, *Nursing Ethics: For Hospital and Private Use* (Cleveland: E.D. Koeckert Publishing, 1912), 38.

8. Ibid.

9. Bertha Harmer, *Textbook of the Principles and Practice of Nursing* (New York: The Macmillan Company, 1922), 3.

10. Scott Hahn and Curtis Mitch, *The Gospel of John* (San Francisco: Ignatius Press, 2003), 45.

11. Neal M. Flanagan, *The Gospel According to John and the Johannine Epistles* (Collegeville, MN: The Liturgical Press, 1989), 62.

12. John J. Pilch, *Galatians and Romans* (Collegeville, MN: The Liturgical Press, 1991).

13. Hannah Hurnard, *Hinds' Feet on High Places* (Wheaton, IL: Tyndale House Publishers, Inc., 1975), 11.

14. Ibid., p. 212.

15. Ibid., pp. 213–214.

16. Kenneth Baker, *Inside the Bible: An Introduction to Each Book of the Bible* (San Francisco: Ignatius Press, 1998), pp. 118–119.

17. David Alexander and Pat Alexander, eds., *Eerdmans Handbook to the Bible* (Grand Rapids, MI: Wm. B. Eerdmans Publishing Co., 1983), 357.

CHAPTER 4: CLOTHED WITH COMPASSION: Entering Sacred Spaces

1. Ivan Havener, *First Thessalonians, Philippians, Philemon, Second Thessalonians, Colossians, Ephesians* (Collegeville, MN: The Liturgical Press, 1991), 78.

2. Ibid.

3. Michael Downey, "Compassion," in *The New Dictionary of Catholic Spirituality,* ed. Michael Downey (Collegeville, MN: The Liturgical Press, 1993), 192–193.

4. Ibid.

5. Ibid.

6. Ibid.

7. Ibid.

8. Mary Breckenridge, *Wide Neighborhoods: A Story of the Frontier Nursing Service* (Lexington, KY: The University Press of Kentucky, 1981).

9. Downey, 192.

10. Florence Nightingale, cited in Joann Widerquist, "Called to Serve," *Christian Nurse International,* 11:1 (1995): 4–6.

11. Joseph Nassal, *The Conspiracy of Compassion: Breathing Together for a Wounded World* (Leavenworth, KS: Forest of Peace Publishing, 1997), 49.

12. Ibid.

13. Richard J. Clifford, *Psalms 1–72* (Collegeville, MN: The Liturgical Press, 1986), p. 51.

14. Algernon Swinburne, "Catherine of Siena," *The Poems of Algernon Charles Swinburne* (London: Chatto and Windus, 1911), 162.

15. Mary A. Nutting and Lavinia L. Dock, *A History of Nursing,* Volumes 1–2 (New York: G.P. Putnam's Sons, 1935), 230.

16. Raymond of Capua, cited in Anne L. Austin, *History of Nursing Sourcebook* (New York: G.P. Putnam's Sons, 1957), 94.

17. James J. Walsh, *The History of Nursing* (New York: P.J. Kenedy & Sons, 1929), 121.

18. Jerome Kodell, *The Gospel According to Luke* (Collegeville, MN: The Liturgical Press, 1989), 52–53.

19. Scott Hahn and Curtis Mitch, *The Gospel of Luke, With Introduction, Commentary and Notes* (San Francisco: Ignatius Press, 2001), 38.

20. David Alexander and Pat Alexander, eds., *Eerdmans Handbook to the Bible* (Grand Rapids, MI: William B. Eerdmans Publishing Co., 1992), 156.

21. Mary Elizabeth O'Brien, *Spirituality in Nursing: Standing on Holy Ground,* 3rd Edition (Sudbury, MA: Jones and Bartlett Publishers, 2007), 1.

22. Jerome Neyrey, *First Timothy, Second Timothy, Titus, James, First Peter, Second Peter, Jude* (Collegeville, MN: The Liturgical Press), 74.

23. John Cardinal O'Connor, *A Moment of Grace: John Cardinal O'Connor on the Catechism of the Catholic Church* (San Francisco: Ignatius Press, 1995), 214.

24. Mary Elizabeth O'Brien, *Prayer in Nursing: The Spirituality of Compassionate Caregiving* (Sudbury, MA: Jones and Bartlett Publishers, 2003), 78–80.

25. Ibid., 82.

26. Neal M. Flanagan, *The Gospel According to John and the Johannine Epistles* (Collegeville, MN: The Liturgical Press, 1989), 47.

CHAPTER 5: WITH STEADFAST DEVOTION: Committed to Caring

1. Mary Elizabeth O'Brien, *Prayer in Nursing: The Spirituality of Compassionate Caregiving* (Sudbury, MA: Jones and Bartlett Publishers, 2003), 12–14.
2. Susan Muto, *Catholic Spirituality From A to Z: An Inspirational Dictionary* (Ann Arbor, MI: Servant Publications, 2000), 68.
3. Francis De Sales, *Introduction to a Devout Life* (New York: Image Books, 1989), 44.
4. Ibid.
5. Monica Baly, ed., *As Miss Nightingale Said... Florence Nightingale Through Her Sayings: A Victorian Perspective* (London: Scutari Press, 1991), 68.
6. William H. Shannon, "Humility," in *The New Dictionary of Catholic Spirituality*, ed. Michael Downey (Collegeville, MN: The Liturgical Press, 1993), 516–518.
7. Ibid.
8. A. H. Lawrence, "To Be A Nurse," cited in Raymond Hain, "Capping Exercises," *The Catholic Nurse* 3:1 (1954): 53–57.
9. "The Nurse's Mass," *The Catholic Nurse* 2:2 (1953): 54–55.
10. Ibid.
11. Ibid.
12. Ibid.
13. Barbara M. Dossey, *Florence Nightingale: Mystic, Visionary, Healer* (Springhouse, PA: Springhouse Corporation, 2000), 33.
14. Mary Elizabeth O'Brien, *The Nurse's Calling: A Christian Spirituality of Caring for the Sick* (Mahwah, NJ: Paulist Press, 2001), 19.
15. Ibid.
16. Hannah Hurnard, *Hinds' Feet on High Places* (Wheaton, IL: Tyndale House Publishers, Inc., 1975).
17. Ibid.
18. Ibid., 63.
19. Mary Clare Vincent, *The Life of Prayer and the Way to God* (Petersham, MA: Saint Bede's Publications, 1982), 1.
20. O'Brien, 2003, 4.
21. Richard J. Cushing, "A Prayer for Nurses," *The Catholic Nurse* 1:2 (1952): 37.
22. "A Nurse's Night Prayer," *The Catholic Nurse* 2:4 (1954): 30–31.

CHAPTER 6: MADE PERFECT IN WEAKNESS: Blessed Vulnerability

1. Carol Picard, "Images of Caring in Nursing and Dance," *Journal of Holistic Nursing* 13:4 (1995): 324–329.

2. Ibid.
3. Scott Hahn and Curtis Mitch, *The Gospel of John* (San Francisco: Ignatius Press), 2003, p. 42.
4. Ibid.
5. Clive S. Lewis, *The Problem of Pain* (New York: The MacMillan Company, 1961), pp. 34–35.
6. Ibid., p. 36.
7. Scott Hahn and Curtis Mitch, *The Gospel of Matthew* (San Francisco: Ignatius Press, 2000), p. 37.
8. Jerome Kodell, *The Gospel According to Luke* (Collegeville, MN: The Liturgical Press, 1989), p. 7.
9. Mary Elizabeth O'Brien, *The Nurse With an Alabaster Jar: A Biblical Approach to Nursing* (Madison, WI: NCF Press, 2006), p. 190.
10. Mary Ann Getty, *First Corinthians, Second Corinthians* (Collegeville, MN: The Liturgical Press, 1991), p. 117.
11. Ibid.
12. Getty, p. 57.
13. Ibid.
14. Kenneth Baker, *Inside the Bible: An Introduction to Each Book of the Bible* (San Francisco: Ignatius Press, 1998), p. 154.
15. Peter Ellis, *Jeremiah, Baruch* (Collegeville, MN: The Liturgical Press, 1986), pp. 64–65.

CHAPTER 7: THE WINTER IS PAST: Empowered by Faith

1. George A. Maloney, *Singers of the New Song: A Mystical Interpretation of the Song of Songs* (Notre Dame, IN: Ave Maria Press, 1985), 52.
2. Ibid.
3. Ibid.
4. Ibid., p. 53.
5. James A. Fischer, *Song of Songs, Ruth, Lamentations, Ecclesiastes, Esther* (Collegeville, MN: The Liturgical Press, 1986), 11.
6. Lawrence Boadt, *Reading the Old Testament: An Introduction* (New York: Paulist Press, 1984), 486.
7. Kenneth Baker, *Inside the Bible: An Introduction to Each Book of the Bible* (San Francisco: Ignatius Press, 1998), 129.
8. John J. Collins, *Isaiah* (Collegeville, MN: The Liturgical Press, 1986), 108.
9. Myra B. Welch, *The Touch of the Master's Hand*, Retrieved December 2, 2006 from www.ehhs.cmich.edu/~tbushey/quote.html
10. Collins, 89.
11. Ibid., 89.

12. Richard J. Clifford, *Psalms 73–150* (Collegeville, MN: The Liturgical Press, 1986), 75.
13. Ibid., 19.
14. John J. Pilch, *Galatians and Romans* (Collegeville, MN: The Liturgical Press, 1991), 61.
15. Ibid., 62.

CHAPTER 8: A DESERTED PLACE: The Mysticism of Everyday Nursing

1. Philip Van Linden, *The Gospel According to Mark* (Collegeville, MN: The Liturgical Press, 1991), 20.
2. Paul J. Achtemeier, "Invitation to Mark," in *Invitation to the Gospels*, eds. Donald Senior, Paul J. Achtemeier, Robert Karris, and George MacRae (Revision by Daniel J. Harrington), (Mahwah, NJ: Paulist Press, 2002), 107–210, 126.
3. Scott Hahn and Curtis Mitch, *The Gospel of Mark* (San Francisco: Ignatius Press, 2001), 19.
4. Richard J. Clifford, *Psalms 1–72* (Collegeville, MN: The Liturgical Press, 1986), 47.
5. Ibid.
6. Kenneth Baker, *Inside the Bible: An Introduction to Each Book of the Bible* (San Francisco: Ignatius Press, 1998), 51.
7. David Alexander and Pat Alexander, eds., *Eerdmans Handbook to the Bible* (Grand Rapids, MI: Wm. B. Eerdmans Publishing Co., 1992), 202.
8. Francis de Sales, "Introduction to a Devout Life," Part II, Chapter 12, cited in Claude Morel, *15 Days of Prayer with Saint Francis de Sales* (Liguori, MO: Liguori, 2000), 33.
9. Brother Lawrence, *The Practice of the Presence of God* (Mount Vernon, NY: Peter Pauper Press, 1973), 48.
10. Brother Roger, *No Greater Love: Sources of Taize* (Collegeville, MN: The Liturgical Press, 1991), 7.
11. Clifford, 46–47.
12. Brother Lawrence of the Resurrection, *The Practice of the Presence of God* (Translated by Robert J. Edmondson) (Brewster, MA: Paraclete Press, 1985), 89–90.
13. Wayne Simsic, *Pray Without Ceasing: Mindfulness of God in Daily Life* (Winona, MN: Saint Mary's Press, 2000), 69.
14. Jan Pettigrew, "Intensive Nursing Care: The Ministry of Presence," *Critical Care Nursing Clinics of North America,* 2:3 (1990), 503–510.
15. Van Linden, 31.
16. Achtemeier, 139.

17. Daniel J. Harrington, *The Gospel According to Matthew* (Collegeville, MN: The Liturgical Press, 1991), 29.

18. Mary Elizabeth O'Brien, *Spirituality in Nursing: Standing on Holy Ground* (Sudbury, MA: Jones and Bartlett Publishers, 2003), 89.

19. Ibid., 99.

20. Mary Ann Getty, *First Corinthians, Second Corinthians* (Collegeville, MN: The Liturgical Press, 1991), 59.

21. Ibid., 60.

22. James A. Wiseman, "Mysticism," in *The New Dictionary of Catholic Spirituality,* ed. Michael Downey (Collegeville, MN: The Liturgical Press, 1993), 681–692.

23. John Welch, "Mysticism," in *The New Dictionary of Theology,* eds. Joseph Komonchak, Mary Collins, and Dermot Lane (Collegeville, MN: The Liturgical Press, 1990), 694–697.

24. Brother Roger of Taize, *His Love Is a Fire* (Collegeville, MN: The Liturgical Press, 1990), 49.

25. Thelma Hall, *Too Deep For Words: Rediscovering Lectio Divina* (Mahwah, NJ: Paulist Press, 1988), 2.

26. Stephen K. Hatch, "The Formation of the Everyday Contemplative," in *The Lay Contemplative: Testimonies, Perspectives, Resources,* eds. Virginia Manss and Mary Frohlich (Cincinnati, OH: St. Anthony Messenger Press, 2000), 59–69.

27. O'Brien, 115.

28. Harvey D. Egan, "The Mysticism of Everyday Life," *Studies in Formative Spirituality,* 10:1 (1989), 8.

29. Ibid.

30. Barbara M. Dossey, Louise C. Selanders, Deva-Marie Beck, and Alex Attewell, *Florence Nightingale Today: Healing, Leadership, Global Action* (Silver Spring, MD: American Nurses Association, 2005), 358.

31. Lynn McDonald, ed., *Florence Nightingale's Spiritual Journey: Biblical Annotations, Sermons and Journal Notes* (Waterloo, Ontario: Wilfrid Laurier University Press, 2001), 77.

32. Lynn McDonald, ed., *Florence Nightingale's Theology: Essay's, Letters and Journal Notes* (Waterloo, Ontario: Wilfrid Laurier University Press, 2001), 232.

33. Gerard Vallee, ed., *Florence Nightingale on Mysticism and Eastern Religions* (Waterloo, Ontario: Wilfrid Laurier University Press, 2001), 20.

34. O'Brien, xiii–xvii.

35. Florence Nightingale, "To Caroline Fleidner, December 1854," cited in Barbara M. Dossey, *Florence Nightingale: Mystic, Visionary, Healer* (Springhouse, PA: Springhouse Corporation, 2000), 121.

Index

Printed in the USA
CPSIA information can be obtained
at www.ICGtesting.com
JSHW010909101123
51570JS00010B/117

9 780763 755713